CKD DIET COOKBOOK:

FOR BEGINNERS, SENIORS AND NEWLY DIAGNOSED

Learn How to Manage Chronic Kidney Disease in All Stages, Prevent Renal Failure and Improve Kidney Functions

Michael Slowick, RDN

COPYRIGHT PAGE

Copyright © 2024 Michael Slowick, RDN. All rights reserved.

No part of this publication or work may be copied, stored in a retrieval system, or transmitted in any form or by any means without prior written permission from the publisher or author, or through payment of the appropriate per-copy fee to the copyright holder, except as permitted under Sections 107 or 108 of the United States Copyright Act of 1976, or as expressly allowed by law, license, or terms agreed upon with the relevant reprographics rights organization.

The publisher and author expressly disclaim any implied guarantees of merchantability and fitness for a particular purpose. While every effort has been made to ensure the accuracy of the information provided herein, no promises are made regarding its completeness or accuracy. Any statements made by sales employees or representatives, whether verbal or written, do not constitute extended or implied guarantees.

Table of Contents

COPYRIGHT PAGE 2

Table of Contents 4

INTRODUCTION 1

CHAPTER I: WHAT DOES CHRONIC KIDNEY DISEASE (CKD) ENTAIL? 1

    Factors contributing to Chronic Kidney Disease 4

    Signs of Chronic Kidney Disease (CKD) 9

CHAPTER II: NUTRITION AND CHRONIC KIDNEY DISEASE 14

    Do you face the possibility of developing Chronic Kidney Disease (CKD)? 20

    Avoiding the Onset of Chronic Kidney Disease 24

    Optimal Nutrition for Chronic Kidney Disease 29

CHAPTER III: CHRONIC KIDNEY DISEASE MANAGEMENT 33

Getting Ready for a Medical Appointment............ 38

Different Renal Conditions... 43

CHAPTER IV: HEALTHFUL, NUTRIENT-DENSE DISHES SUITABLE FOR KIDNEY HEALTH............. 48

KIDNEY-SUPPORTIVE MORNING MEAL IDEAS. 48

    Arugula Salad... 48

    Breakfast Strata... 49

    Overnight Eggnog French Toast............................... 52

    Sausage Egg Muffins 54

    Cheesy Bacon, Sausage, and Egg Hash Brown Skillet 56

    Peanut Butter and Jelly French Toast Casserole.... 59

    Overnight Breakfast Bake with Ham, Cheese, and Croissants 62

    Dash's Donair... 65

    Chilaquiles 68

Chicken Caesar Wrap 70

Greek Island Chicken Shish Kebabs 72

Briam (Greek Baked Zucchini and Potatoes) 74

Zucchini Artichoke Summer Salad 76

Avocado and Tuna Tapas 78

KIDNEY-FRIENDLY NOONTIME MEAL IDEAS ... 83

Scallops Provencale 83

Marinated Green Beans with Olives, Tomatoes, and Feta 85

Pan-Seared Scallops with Pepper and Onions in Anchovy Oil 87

Braised Chicken and Artichoke Hearts with Lemon, Cherry Peppers and Thyme 90

Insalata Caprese 92

Cucumber Sandwiches 93

Spiced Sweet Roasted Red Pepper Hummus 96

Lemon Chicken Piccata 97

Broiled Spanish Mackerel 100

Fried Soft-Shell Crab.. 102

Pan-Seared Salmon 104

Capers and Halibut... 106

Spanish Moroccan Fish 107

Nicoise-Style Tuna Salad With White Beans & Olives 110

Cucumber Gazpacho 112

KIDNEY-SUPPORTIVE SUPPER IDEAS 115

Garlic Escargots... 115

Oven Roasted Red Potatoes and Asparagus........ 117

Dutch Apple Pie with Oatmeal Streusel............... 119

Baked Mac and Cheese with Sour Cream and Cottage Cheese 122

Baked Feta Cheese and Tomatoes 124

Tuna Casserole 127

Balsamic Grilled Zucchini 128

Italian Rice Balls 129

Mushroom Rice 132

Grilled Pattypan Squash With Garlic Butter 133

Crisp Pickled Green Beans 135

Sausage Stuffed Jalapeños 138

Stuffed Pork Chops 139

'Chinese Buffet' Green Beans 141

Asparagus Wrapped in Crisp Prosciutto 143

KIDNEY-FRIENDLY SOUP RECIPES 144

Chilled Corn Soup 144

Roasted Carrot and Tahini Soup 146

Bone Broth 149

Spinach Artichoke Soup 151

Roasted Apple and Parsnip Soup 153

Stracciatella Soup 155

Feta Shrimp Soup 157

Zucchini Fenchel Suppe (Zucchini and Fennel Soup) 159

Italian Sausage Soup 161

Spanish Garlic Soup 162

Asparagus, Lemon, and Mint Soup 164

Fresh Asparagus Soup 166

Southwestern Turkey Soup 169

Coconut Black Bean Soup 171

Cheeseburger Soup 172

KIDNEY-SUPPORTIVE SWEET TREAT IDEAS 175

Lava Cake 175

Quiche Lorraine 177

Mini Pecan Pies 179

Meringues 181

Little Nut Cups 182

Bologna Sliders with Fried Onions 185

Baked Pumpkin Custard 186

Cranberry Brie Bites 188

Grilled Hot Dog Sliders 191

Butter Tarts 192

Pepperoni Pizza Muffins 193

Red Lobster Cheddar Biscuits 195

Cake Pops 198

Red, White, and Blue Cheesecake Bites 201

Baked Ham and Cheese Sliders 205

CHAPTER V: FINAL NOTES 208

INTRODUCTION

Welcome to the comprehensive guide on Chronic Kidney Disease (CKD) and its dietary management. This book is designed to provide invaluable insights and practical strategies for individuals navigating the complex terrain of CKD and its impact on dietary choices.

Chronic Kidney Disease is a prevalent and serious condition affecting millions of people worldwide. Characterized by the gradual loss of kidney function over time, CKD necessitates meticulous attention to various aspects of daily life, including diet and nutrition.

You possess a pair of kidneys, bean-shaped organs positioned towards your back on either side of your spine, just beneath your rib cage, each roughly the size of your fist.

The primary function of your kidneys is to purify your blood by eliminating toxins, waste, and excess water as urine. Additionally, they regulate electrolyte and mineral levels, produce hormones controlling blood pressure, generate red blood cells, and maintain bone strength. Should your kidneys sustain damage and function improperly, toxins may accumulate in your bloodstream, causing illness.

Chronic kidney disease, or chronic kidney failure, denotes a gradual decline in kidney function. Initially, your kidneys filter waste and surplus fluids from your blood, excreting them in urine. However, advanced chronic kidney disease can lead to dangerous levels of fluid, electrolytes, and waste accumulation in your body.

During the early stages of chronic kidney disease, symptoms may be minimal or absent, with the condition often remaining undetected until it progresses.

Treatment for chronic kidney disease aims to retard kidney damage progression, typically by managing the underlying cause. However, controlling the cause may not always prevent kidney damage from worsening. If untreated, chronic kidney disease can advance to end-stage kidney failure, necessitating artificial filtration (dialysis) or a kidney transplant for survival.

In chronic kidney disease, kidney function gradually diminishes, with lasting damage that can exacerbate over time, progressing through various stages. While anyone can develop CKD, certain demographics, such as older individuals and those of South Asian or Black descent, are at higher risk.

Chronic kidney disease, also known as chronic renal disease, signifies kidney damage leading to diminished function. The kidneys act as a filtration system, removing waste, toxins, and excess water from the blood, while also supporting bone and red blood cell health.

As kidney function declines, waste accumulates in the blood, contributing to the chronic nature of the disease. CKD can culminate in kidney failure, also termed end-stage kidney disease.

Although not all CKD patients progress to kidney failure, the condition typically worsens without intervention. While there is no cure for chronic kidney disease, strategies exist to decelerate kidney damage.

Dialysis and transplantation are viable options for end-stage kidney disease.

CHAPTER I: WHAT DOES CHRONIC KIDNEY DISEASE (CKD) ENTAIL?

When your kidneys sustain damage severe enough to impair their ability to adequately filter your blood, it leads to a condition known as chronic kidney disease (CKD). This isn't just a simple malfunction; it's a complex cascade of events that can have profound and long-lasting effects on your health.

Picture your kidneys as meticulous janitors stationed in the lower part of your back, diligently sifting through every drop of blood that courses through your body. Their job is to meticulously remove waste products and excess water, leaving behind a purified stream of blood ready to nourish your organs and tissues. But when these vital organs are compromised, this delicate process is disrupted, leading to a buildup of toxins and waste materials in your bloodstream. This accumulation isn't just a nuisance; it can trigger a domino effect of health issues that span far beyond the confines of your kidneys.

Beyond their role as blood purifiers, kidneys also serve as master regulators of your body's mineral balance. They carefully orchestrate the levels of essential minerals like calcium, phosphorus, sodium, and potassium, ensuring that everything stays in perfect harmony. Additionally, they moonlight as hormone factories, churning out substances that play pivotal roles in maintaining your cardiovascular health, supporting blood cell formation, and even safeguarding your bone density.

But when chronic kidney disease sets in, it's like throwing a wrench into a finely tuned machine.

Suddenly, this intricate balance is thrown off-kilter, setting the stage for a host of complications. Long-term kidney dysfunction isn't just a minor inconvenience; it significantly heightens your risk of progressing to kidney failure, a dire scenario where your kidneys can no longer keep up with the demands of your body.

In the face of kidney failure, the options become stark: either undergo the rigors of dialysis, where a machine takes on the role of your faltering kidneys, or brave the uncertainties of a kidney transplant, hoping to find a suitable donor match. These interventions aren't just medical procedures; they're lifelines, offering a chance at survival in the face of overwhelming odds.

But here's the glimmer of hope amidst the gloom: kidney disease, if detected early, can often be effectively managed and treated. Like any formidable opponent, the key lies in early detection and proactive intervention. By keeping a vigilant eye on your kidney health and heeding the warning signs, you can tilt the odds in your favor, potentially staving off the worst consequences of this silent but insidious condition.

Factors contributing to Chronic Kidney Disease

Chronic kidney failure (CKD) stands as a significant health concern, with its primary culprits often identified as diabetes and hypertension. These conditions, with their insidious progression, can silently wreak havoc on renal function, leading to a cascade of complications if left unchecked.

When grappling with kidney issues, the journey to diagnosis involves a thorough exploration of one's medical history and possibly an array of diagnostic tests orchestrated by a vigilant healthcare provider. Unraveling the mystery behind renal ailments demands a meticulous approach, considering the myriad factors that could be at play.

Let's delve into the intricacies of these two chief instigators of CKD: diabetes and hypertension. Diabetes, characterized by elevated levels of glucose in the bloodstream, can inflict considerable damage on the delicate filtration mechanism of the kidneys over time. The insidious nature of this metabolic disorder gradually impairs the kidneys' ability to rid the body of waste products and excess fluids. One of the earliest red flags of diabetes-related kidney impairment is the presence of protein, notably albumin, in the urine—a telltale sign of compromised renal function. Such manifestations underscore the gravity of what's clinically termed as diabetic kidney disease, a condition that demands prompt attention and tailored interventions.

Meanwhile, hypertension, or high blood pressure, emerges as another formidable adversary in the realm of renal health. The relentless force exerted by elevated blood pressure levels exacts a toll on the intricate network of blood vessels nourishing the kidneys. This vascular assault impedes the kidneys' vital task of waste removal and fluid regulation, setting off a vicious cycle of dysfunction. As fluid accumulates within the bloodstream, blood pressure surges further, exacerbating the strain on already beleaguered renal arteries. The repercussions of uncontrolled hypertension on renal integrity serve as a stark reminder of the interconnectedness between cardiovascular health and kidney function.

However, the plot thickens as we unravel the myriad other factors capable of precipitating kidney maladies. Hereditary predispositions rear their head in conditions like polycystic kidney disease (PKD), where cyst formation runs rampant within the renal parenchyma, spelling trouble for renal function. Infections, too, can incite renal havoc, triggering a cascade of inflammatory responses that jeopardize renal integrity. Furthermore, nefarious substances masquerading as therapeutic agents—think nephrotoxic drugs—can inflict renal injury if wielded recklessly, underscoring the importance of judicious medication management.

The realm of systemic diseases casts a wide net of influence over renal health, with conditions like diabetes and lupus showcasing renal involvement as one of their cardinal manifestations. The ominous specter of autoimmune disorders, exemplified by anti-

GBM (Goodpasture's) disease, serves as a poignant reminder of the body's propensity to turn against its own tissues, including the kidneys. Heavy metal poisoning, albeit rare, lurks as a lurking threat to renal well-being, particularly in environments tainted by the toxic presence of lead.

Moreover, the genetic lottery can deal a cruel hand in the form of rare disorders such as Alport syndrome, where genetic aberrations conspire to undermine renal structure and function. Even seemingly innocuous childhood illnesses like Hemolytic Uremic Syndrome can leave a lasting imprint on renal health, underscoring the vulnerability of young kidneys to external assaults.

The tapestry of renal diseases extends beyond the confines of common knowledge, weaving a complex narrative that demands a holistic understanding of the myriad factors at play. From the microscopic realm of molecular aberrations to the macroscopic landscape of environmental exposures, every facet of our existence holds sway over the delicate balance of renal health. In navigating this labyrinthine landscape, vigilance, education, and proactive healthcare engagement emerge as our steadfast allies in safeguarding the precious gift of renal well-being.

Signs of Chronic Kidney Disease (CKD)

Recognizing the early signs of Chronic Kidney Disease (CKD) can be elusive, as symptoms may not always manifest conspicuously. It's not uncommon for individuals to feel relatively well despite underlying CKD, a phenomenon that can perplex onlookers. Remarkably, the kidneys possess an extraordinary capacity to perform their vital functions, often surpassing mere survival requirements.

Contrary to common misconceptions, the act of donating a kidney does not inherently jeopardize one's prospects for leading a healthy and fulfilling life. Even in the presence of kidney impairment, many individuals continue to carry out their daily activities without significant hindrance. Diagnosis of kidney disease often hinges upon meticulous blood and urine tests, serving as primary diagnostic tools for healthcare professionals.

As renal disease progresses, manifestations such as edema, characterized by swelling, may emerge. This swelling results from the kidneys' diminished ability to effectively filter excess fluid and salt from the body. Notably, edema can affect various parts of the body, including the hands, face, and lower extremities, further highlighting the systemic impact of renal dysfunction.

The spectrum of symptoms associated with advanced CKD is diverse and can significantly impact an individual's quality of life. From chest discomfort to dry skin, itching, numbness, and profound fatigue, the array of potential symptoms underscores the multifaceted nature of this condition. Furthermore, changes in urine frequency, loss of appetite, muscular cramps, nausea, shortness of breath, sleep disturbances, difficulty concentrating, vomiting, and weight loss may all signal the progression of CKD. Importantly, chronic kidney disease patients also face heightened risks of anemia, skeletal issues, and malnutrition, compounding the complexity of managing their health.

Beyond its direct physiological implications, CKD poses a substantial risk factor for cardiovascular disease, heightening the likelihood of strokes and heart attacks among affected individuals. Hypertension, a common comorbidity of CKD, not only exacerbates renal dysfunction but also predisposes individuals to kidney damage. The intricate interplay between hypertension and kidney health underscores the importance of comprehensive management strategies in mitigating the progression of CKD and its associated complications.

Furthermore, individuals with CKD face heightened susceptibility to abrupt fluctuations in kidney function triggered by illness, injury, or certain medications, a condition referred to as Acute Kidney Injury (AKI). This underscores the importance of diligent monitoring and proactive management strategies to safeguard kidney health and mitigate the risk of acute complications.

The nuanced manifestations of CKD underscore the complexity of renal health management, necessitating a multifaceted approach encompassing early detection, diligent monitoring, and comprehensive intervention strategies to optimize outcomes and enhance quality of life for affected individuals.

CHAPTER II: NUTRITION AND CHRONIC KIDNEY DISEASE

Ensuring the prevention of waste accumulation within the bloodstream becomes paramount for individuals grappling with compromised kidney function. This necessitates strict adherence to a renal or kidney diet, carefully curated to mitigate the influx of waste products derived from food and beverages. When the intricate filtration mechanism of the kidneys falters, the efficiency in waste removal diminishes, resulting in a retention of toxins within the body.

The repercussions of this impaired waste clearance extend to the delicate balance of electrolytes within the system. Elevated levels of waste compounds in the blood can disrupt electrolyte equilibrium, potentially instigating adverse physiological effects. Therefore, preserving kidney health and staving off the progression toward renal failure hinges significantly on dietary interventions tailored to address these concerns.

Central to the renal diet regimen is the regulation of sodium, phosphorus, and protein intake. This entails not only curtailing the consumption of these elements but also embracing dietary strategies that promote optimal kidney function. Moreover, considerations extend to fluid management, recognizing the pivotal role of hydration in renal health.

Navigating the nuances of a renal diet necessitates individualized attention, acknowledging the unique nutritional requirements of each person. Collaboration with a renal dietician emerges as indispensable in crafting a bespoke dietary plan that aligns with one's specific needs and health status. Understanding the broader context of a renal diet, it becomes evident that several key metrics warrant diligent monitoring and management.

Sodium, a ubiquitous mineral ingrained in various foodstuffs, assumes a critical role in bodily functions spanning from blood pressure regulation to nerve transmission. However, individuals grappling with renal impairment confront heightened susceptibility to sodium-induced complications, necessitating vigilant control over its intake. Strategies encompass scrutinizing food labels, opting for fresh produce, and eschewing processed fare to curtail sodium consumption effectively.

Likewise, potassium, another essential electrolyte integral to cardiac and muscular function, demands meticulous oversight in the renal diet landscape. As renal dysfunction compromises potassium excretion, its accumulation can precipitate grave cardiovascular repercussions. Managing potassium intake involves strategic meal planning and judicious selection of potassium-rich foods, under the guidance of a healthcare professional.

Phosphorus, revered for its role in skeletal health and cellular function, presents another facet of concern in renal dietary management. Excessive phosphorus levels, stemming from impaired renal filtration, pose a dual threat of bone demineralization and cardiovascular compromise. Mitigating phosphorus overload necessitates vigilance in food selection, opting for low-phosphorus alternatives, and leveraging dietary interventions to circumvent its accumulation.

Furthermore, protein, a dietary staple pivotal for tissue repair and metabolic processes, warrants nuanced adjustment in the renal diet paradigm. Balancing protein intake becomes imperative to forestall the accumulation of metabolic waste products, which kidneys struggle to excrete efficiently in compromised states. Thus, adhering to personalized protein recommendations emerges as a cornerstone in preserving renal function and overall well-being.

Fluid management assumes added significance in the realm of renal dietary considerations, particularly for individuals navigating advanced stages of chronic kidney disease (CKD) or undergoing dialysis. Striking a delicate equilibrium in fluid intake becomes imperative to avert complications stemming from fluid overload, including cardiovascular strain and pulmonary distress. Adherence to tailored fluid intake guidelines, guided by medical professionals, constitutes a pivotal aspect of renal diet adherence.

The intricate interplay between dietary constituents and renal health underscores the significance of a meticulously tailored renal diet regimen. By embracing dietary modifications encompassing sodium, potassium, phosphorus, protein, and fluid intake, individuals can proactively mitigate the progression of renal dysfunction and foster optimal well-being. This collaborative endeavor, underpinned by the expertise of healthcare professionals, empowers individuals to navigate the complexities of renal dietary management with confidence and efficacy.

Do you face the possibility of developing Chronic Kidney Disease (CKD)?

Chronic kidney disease (CKD) affects a significant portion of the United States population, with estimates indicating that more than 37 million individuals are currently grappling with this condition. It's a complex health concern with multifaceted origins and impacts.

One of the primary culprits behind CKD is diabetes, a condition that affects numerous Americans. Shockingly, nearly one-third of individuals diagnosed with diabetes will eventually find themselves contending with CKD. This linkage stems from the detrimental effects of elevated blood glucose levels, which wreak havoc on the delicate blood vessels within the kidneys, ultimately leading to chronic damage and dysfunction.

Following closely behind diabetes as a leading cause of CKD is high blood pressure. Studies have revealed that approximately one-fifth of individuals living with hypertension will develop CKD, underscoring the significant role that hypertension plays in renal health. Just like with diabetes, the persistent elevation of blood pressure can inflict substantial harm on the renal blood vessels, exacerbating the risk of kidney disease.

The intricate interplay between renal health and cardiovascular wellness further complicates matters. Research has shown that individuals already grappling with kidney issues face an elevated risk of developing heart disease, highlighting the interconnected nature of these vital bodily systems. Scientists are diligently delving into this complex relationship to unravel the underlying mechanisms and identify potential avenues for intervention and prevention.

Moreover, familial predispositions play a notable role in the development of CKD. Having a family member who has experienced kidney failure significantly heightens one's susceptibility to the disease, emphasizing the importance of proactive testing and monitoring among relatives, especially during celebratory gatherings and family reunions.

Age and a medical history rife with chronic conditions such as diabetes, hypertension, or cardiovascular disease serve as additional risk factors for CKD. These factors compound the likelihood of developing kidney disease, underscoring the importance of comprehensive health management and preventive care strategies.

Furthermore, disparities in CKD prevalence among different racial and ethnic groups demand attention and investigation. People of color, particularly African Americans, Hispanics, and American Indians, are disproportionately affected by CKD, primarily due to the higher incidence rates of diabetes and hypertension within these communities. While these factors contribute to the heightened risk, ongoing research endeavors strive to uncover additional explanations for this disparity, aiming to address and mitigate health inequities.

Amidst this complex landscape, dietary modifications emerge as a crucial tool in the prevention and management of renal disease. Adopting a balanced and nutritious diet tailored to individual health needs can help mitigate risk factors and promote kidney health, offering a proactive approach to safeguarding against the onset and progression of CKD.

Chronic kidney disease represents a significant public health challenge, with its origins intertwined with prevalent conditions like diabetes and hypertension, compounded by familial predispositions and demographic disparities. Understanding the multifaceted nature of CKD and implementing comprehensive preventive measures, including dietary interventions, is essential in addressing this pervasive health concern and improving outcomes for individuals at risk.

Avoiding the Onset of Chronic Kidney Disease

Incorporating physical activity into your daily routine is vital for maintaining overall health and well-being. Aim to carve out time each day, even if it's just a brief window, to engage in some form of exercise. Striving for at least 30 minutes of moderate exercise most days of the week can significantly benefit your physical and mental health.

If you're not currently active, it's wise to consult with your healthcare provider to determine the most suitable types of exercise and duration for your individual needs and abilities. They can offer tailored recommendations based on your health status and any underlying medical conditions you may have.

Embarking on a journey toward a more active lifestyle requires commitment and guidance. Consider exploring various strategies to incorporate more movement into your daily life. This might involve scheduling regular walks, joining fitness classes, or discovering enjoyable recreational activities that get you moving.

Maintaining a healthy weight is also crucial for overall health. If you're carrying excess weight or are concerned about your weight, discussing your options with a healthcare professional or registered nutritionist can provide valuable insights and support. They can assist you in developing a personalized plan to achieve and sustain a weight that is optimal for your health.

Ensuring adequate sleep is another cornerstone of well-being. Aim for 7 to 8 hours of quality sleep each night by establishing a consistent bedtime routine. If you struggle with sleep disturbances, consider implementing relaxation techniques or seeking guidance to address underlying factors contributing to sleep difficulties.

For individuals who smoke or use tobacco products, quitting is a significant step toward improving health outcomes. Don't hesitate to seek support from healthcare professionals, support groups, or cessation programs to increase your chances of success.

Moderating alcohol consumption is also important for overall health. Excessive alcohol intake can have adverse effects on various aspects of health, including blood pressure regulation and weight management. If you choose to drink alcohol, do so in moderation, adhering to recommended limits.

Exploring relaxation techniques can further enhance your overall well-being. Practices such as meditation, yoga, tai chi, and deep breathing exercises can help alleviate stress and promote relaxation. Additionally, integrating regular physical activity into your routine can serve as a natural stress reliever and mood enhancer.

For individuals managing chronic kidney disease (CKD), dietary modifications may be necessary to optimize kidney function and prevent complications. Your healthcare provider may recommend reducing phosphorus and potassium intake to maintain optimal blood levels. Familiarize yourself with foods that are lower in phosphorus and potassium and consider working with a dietitian to develop a customized meal plan.

Incorporating phosphate binders into your regimen as prescribed by your healthcare provider can help control phosphorus levels and reduce the risk of complications associated with CKD. Additionally, being mindful of potassium-rich foods and avoiding excessive salt substitutes can help maintain electrolyte balance and support kidney health.

By prioritizing physical activity, healthy eating, adequate sleep, tobacco cessation, alcohol moderation, stress management, and kidney-friendly dietary practices, you can take proactive steps toward optimizing your overall health and well-being. Remember, small changes can lead to significant improvements in your quality of life over time.

Optimal Nutrition for Chronic Kidney Disease

Many individuals opt for a balanced diet that includes both plant- and animal-based foods due to the fact that each offers valuable protein content essential for bodily functions. Consulting with a qualified nutritionist can provide personalized guidance on incorporating optimal protein-rich options into one's dietary regimen.

Animal-derived protein sources encompass a variety of options such as chicken, fish, meat, eggs, and dairy products. Typically, a standard serving size of cooked animal protein ranges from 2 to 3 ounces, akin to the dimensions of a standard deck of playing cards. Meanwhile, dairy servings equate to about half a cup of milk, yogurt, or cheese.

On the other hand, plant-based protein sources encompass a diverse array of choices including beans, nuts, and grains. A half-cup of cooked beans constitutes a serving, while a quarter cup of nuts is considered equivalent to one serving. Similarly, a single piece of bread constitutes a serving, and half a cup of cooked rice or noodles is also deemed as one serving.

Prioritizing heart-friendly food choices is paramount to ward off the accumulation of unhealthy fats within the body's arteries, organs, and circulatory system. Opting for cooking methods like grilling, broiling, baking, roasting, or stir-frying over deep frying can significantly reduce the intake of excess fats. Furthermore, substituting butter with nonstick cooking spray or a dash of olive oil during meal preparation offers a healthier alternative.

Moreover, conscientiously trimming excess fat from meat and removing poultry skin prior to cooking or consumption can further mitigate the intake of unhealthy fats. Diligently reading food labels aids in identifying and limiting the consumption of saturated and trans fats, thus promoting cardiovascular health.

In terms of dietary choices conducive to heart health, options such as lean cuts of meat like loin and round, skinless chicken, fish, legumes, vegetables, fruits, and low-fat or fat-free dairy products like milk, yogurt, and cheese are highly recommended. By incorporating these nutritious selections into one's daily meals, individuals can proactively support their cardiovascular well-being and overall health.

CHAPTER III: CHRONIC KIDNEY DISEASE MANAGEMENT

Ensuring the protection and preservation of kidney function is paramount for individuals living with Chronic Kidney Disease (CKD). Taking proactive steps to mitigate the risk of further kidney damage not only safeguards renal health but also diminishes the likelihood of developing cardiovascular complications and enhances overall well-being. This proactive approach remains imperative even in the absence of overt symptoms, underscoring the importance of early intervention and preventive strategies.

To effectively safeguard against kidney disease progression, a multifaceted approach is warranted. Firstly, maintaining optimal blood pressure levels is crucial, as hypertension exacerbates renal deterioration. Individuals with diabetes must diligently manage their blood sugar levels to minimize the strain on the kidneys. Regular monitoring of kidney function through collaborative efforts with healthcare providers facilitates timely intervention and personalized treatment plans. Adherence to prescribed medication regimens is imperative to forestall exacerbation of kidney damage.

Nutritional interventions play a pivotal role in kidney health maintenance. Consulting with a registered dietitian to develop a tailored dietary plan ensures adequate nourishment while mitigating stress on renal function. Embracing a dietary pattern rich in whole grains, fruits, vegetables, and lean proteins fosters cardiovascular health and supports renal function. Limiting salt intake, reducing consumption of processed foods, and moderating sugar intake are integral components of a kidney-friendly diet. Furthermore, incorporating healthy cooking methods and mindful eating practices optimize nutritional intake and promote satiety.

Regular physical activity is indispensable in mitigating the risk of kidney disease progression and fostering overall health. Engaging in regular exercise routines supports cardiovascular health, regulates blood pressure, and promotes weight management. Adequate sleep hygiene and stress management techniques are instrumental in mitigating the adverse effects of chronic conditions on renal health. Cessation of tobacco use and adoption of healthy coping mechanisms alleviate the burden on the kidneys and mitigate the risk of complications.

Individuals with diabetes must maintain vigilant surveillance of blood sugar levels to optimize glycemic control and minimize the risk of renal complications. Regular monitoring of hemoglobin A1C levels provides insight into long-term blood glucose management and informs therapeutic interventions. Collaborating closely with healthcare providers to establish individualized glycemic targets and treatment goals optimizes renal health outcomes.

In addition to glycemic control, managing comorbidities such as urinary tract infections (UTIs) is paramount in preserving renal function. Timely detection and treatment of UTIs prevent progression to more severe renal complications, safeguarding kidney health.

Adhering to a heart-healthy dietary pattern, such as the Dietary Approaches to Stop Hypertension (DASH) diet, confers benefits beyond blood pressure management. Embracing dietary modifications aimed at reducing sodium intake, increasing consumption of fruits, vegetables, and whole grains, and limiting saturated fats promotes renal health and mitigates cardiovascular risk factors.

In conclusion, prioritizing preventive measures and adopting a holistic approach to kidney health maintenance are essential in mitigating the progression of CKD and safeguarding overall well-being. By implementing proactive strategies encompassing lifestyle modifications, regular monitoring, and disease management, individuals can optimize renal function and mitigate the risk of adverse outcomes associated with kidney disease.

Getting Ready for a Medical Appointment

Taking an active role in preparing for your doctor's visits can significantly enhance your understanding of your health and treatment options. Instead of relying solely on your doctor's guidance, you can empower yourself by creating a comprehensive list of questions and concerns. This proactive approach ensures that no important aspect of your health goes unaddressed during your appointments.

When compiling your list of questions, it's essential to jot down any inquiries that arise, no matter how trivial they may seem at the moment. Questions about the tests you undergo, the significance of their results, and potential dietary or pharmaceutical adjustments should all find a place on your list. By systematically organizing your concerns, you can ensure that you cover all pertinent topics during your appointment.

For individuals grappling with kidney illness, a sample set of questions can serve as a helpful starting point. These questions may encompass various aspects of kidney health, such as glomerular filtration rate (GFR), albumin levels in urine, and the progression of renal disease. Additionally, inquiries about blood pressure readings and potential treatment interventions can provide valuable insights into managing the condition effectively.

Beyond medical queries, considerations about medical care, personal hygiene, and potential difficulties should also be addressed. Patients may seek guidance on preventing the exacerbation of their condition, adjusting medication regimens, adhering to dietary recommendations, and accessing specialized care from nephrologists or dieticians. Furthermore, discussing potential complications and early warning signs can empower patients to take proactive measures in safeguarding their health.

Navigating medical appointments can be daunting, but having a trusted companion by your side can provide invaluable support. Whether it's a family member or friend, their presence can facilitate communication, offer emotional reassurance, and help retain important information shared during the appointment. Prior communication with your companion about your expectations and desired level of involvement can ensure a fruitful collaboration during the visit.

In the realm of healthcare, collaboration among various professionals is paramount in delivering comprehensive care. Your treatment team may consist of diverse healthcare providers, each playing a distinct role in managing your condition. From primary care providers and registered nurses to dieticians and pharmacists, each member contributes expertise tailored to your specific needs.

Maintaining open communication with your healthcare team is essential, particularly regarding medication management. As kidney function fluctuates, adjustments to medication regimens may be necessary to optimize treatment outcomes and minimize adverse effects. Patients are encouraged to disclose all medications, including over-the-counter supplements, to their healthcare providers to mitigate potential drug interactions and complications.

In addition to medication management, attention to over-the-counter medications warrants caution, particularly nonsteroidal anti-inflammatory drugs (NSAIDs). These medications, commonly used for pain relief and fever reduction, can inadvertently exacerbate kidney damage if used indiscriminately. Patients are advised to consult with their healthcare providers regarding the safety and appropriateness of over-the-counter medications.

Furthermore, dietary considerations play a pivotal role in managing kidney disease. Collaborating with a registered dietitian can facilitate the development of a personalized nutrition plan that aligns with your health goals and preferences. Medical nutrition therapy, often covered by insurance for individuals with chronic conditions like diabetes or renal disease, offers tailored dietary guidance to optimize health outcomes.

Incorporating regular exercise into your routine complements dietary and medical interventions in managing kidney disease. Physical activity not only promotes overall well-being but also contributes to stress reduction, weight management, and the attainment of blood pressure and blood glucose targets. Patients are encouraged to discuss suitable exercise regimens with their healthcare providers to ensure safe and effective participation.

Proactive engagement in healthcare decision-making empowers patients to actively participate in their treatment journey. By arming themselves with knowledge, asking pertinent questions, and fostering collaboration with their healthcare team, individuals can optimize their health outcomes and quality of life despite facing challenges posed by kidney disease.

Different Renal Conditions

A simple renal cyst, medically termed as such, represents a benign condition characterized by the formation of fluid-filled sacs within the kidneys. These cysts may occur singularly or in clusters and can vary in size from as small as a pea to as large as a golf ball, typically assuming a rounded or oval shape.

Distinguishing them from conditions like polycystic kidney disease (PKD), a hereditary disorder associated with chronic kidney dysfunction, simple kidney cysts generally pose no threat to kidney size, structure, or function. Predominantly observed in older individuals, particularly men who exhibit twice the propensity compared to women, these cysts tend to augment in prevalence and magnitude with advancing age.

Though often asymptomatic and devoid of significant health implications, larger cysts may manifest symptoms such as localized pain due to compression of adjacent structures, obstruction of urinary flow, infection leading to discomfort or complications, rupture resulting in hematuria, or even provocation of hypertension.

While the majority of simple kidney cysts are incidentally detected during unrelated diagnostic imaging, further evaluation may be warranted to rule out underlying malignancies such as certain types of kidney cancer. However, upon confirmation of a simple cyst, additional intervention or treatment is seldom necessary, unless warranted by symptomatic or complicating factors.

In instances where cysts reach considerable dimensions, surgical intervention may be indicated. Typically performed under general anesthesia within a hospital setting, the procedure involves drainage of the cyst followed by excision or cauterization of surrounding tissue. Recovery generally necessitates a brief hospital stay spanning one to two days.

Switching gears to nephrolithiasis, commonly known as kidney stones, these solid formations arise from the precipitation of minerals within the urinary tract, often due to elevated concentrations in the urine. Varying in size from minuscule to considerably large, kidney stones can provoke excruciating pain and complications if they obstruct urinary flow.

Presenting in diverse compositions including calcium oxalate, calcium phosphate, uric acid, struvite, and cystine, each type of kidney stone is associated with distinct causative factors and preventive measures. Strategies to mitigate the risk of stone formation typically revolve around adequate hydration to maintain urine dilution and modification of dietary habits based on stone composition.

Furthermore, kidney infections, stemming primarily from bacterial or viral invasion of the urinary tract, can lead to severe complications if left untreated. While the body's innate defenses typically ward off urinary tract infections, failure of these mechanisms can precipitate the ascent of pathogens to the kidneys, culminating in potentially life-threatening conditions necessitating prompt medical intervention.

While renal cysts, kidney stones, and urinary tract infections represent disparate entities, they collectively underscore the importance of vigilant monitoring, prompt diagnosis, and appropriate management to safeguard renal health and avert potential complications.

CHAPTER IV: HEALTHFUL, NUTRIENT-DENSE DISHES SUITABLE FOR KIDNEY HEALTH

KIDNEY-SUPPORTIVE MORNING MEAL IDEAS

Arugula Salad

What You Need

4 cups young arugula leaves, rinsed and dried

1 cup cherry tomatoes, halved

¼ cup pine nuts

¼ cup grated Parmesan cheese

2 tablespoons grapeseed or olive oil

1 tablespoon rice vinegar

salt and freshly ground black pepper to taste

1 large avocado - peeled, pitted, and sliced

Instructions

Combine arugula, tomatoes, pine nuts, Parmesan, oil, and vinegar in a large, lidded plastic bowl. Season with salt and pepper, then cover with the lid and shake to mix.

Divide salad onto serving plates and top with avocado slices.

Breakfast Strata

What You Need

1 pound sausage, casings removed

2 cups sliced fresh mushrooms

8 eggs, beaten

10 cups cubed, day-old bread

3 cups whole milk

2 cups shredded Cheddar cheese

1 ½ cups cubed Black Forest ham

1 (10 ounce) package frozen chopped spinach, thawed and drained

2 tablespoons all-purpose flour

2 tablespoons mustard powder

1 teaspoon salt

2 teaspoons butter, melted

2 teaspoons dried basil

Instructions

Generously grease a 9x13-inch casserole dish.

Heat a skillet over medium heat; cook and stir sausage until crumbly and completely browned, about 10 minutes. Transfer cooked sausage to the prepared casserole dish.

Cook and stir mushrooms in the same skillet over medium heat until liquid has been released and mushrooms are lightly browned, 5 to 10 minutes; drain.

Mix mushrooms, eggs, bread, milk, Cheddar cheese, ham, spinach, flour, mustard powder, salt, butter, and basil together in a large bowl; pour over sausage. Cover casserole dish and refrigerate, 2 hours to overnight.

Preheat oven to 350 degrees F (175 degrees C).

Bake in the preheated oven until a knife inserted into the center of the strata comes out clean, 60 to 70 minutes.

Overnight Eggnog French Toast

What You Need

1 cup brown sugar

½ cup butter

2 tablespoons light corn syrup

1 loaf French bread, cut into 1-inch slices

8 eggs

2 cups prepared eggnog

Instructions

Lightly grease a 9x13-inch baking dish.

Heat the brown sugar, butter, and corn syrup in a small saucepan over medium heat. Cook and stir until the mixture begins to boil; remove the mixture from heat, and pour into the prepared baking dish. Place the bread slices atop the brown sugar mixture.

Whisk the eggs and eggnog together in a large bowl; pour over the bread slices. Cover the baking dish with aluminum foil, and refrigerate 8 hours to overnight.

Preheat an oven to 325 degrees F (165 degrees C). Remove the baking dish from the refrigerator.

Bake in the preheated oven for 35 minutes. Increase heat to 375 degrees F (190 degrees C), remove the aluminum foil, and continue baking until the the top begins to brown, 5 to 7 minutes more.

Sausage Egg Muffins

What You Need

½ pound ground pork sausage

12 large eggs, beaten

1 small onion, chopped

½ (4 ounce) can chopped green chile peppers, drained

1 teaspoon garlic powder

salt and pepper to taste

Instructions

Preheat the oven to 350 degrees F (175 degrees C). Lightly grease a 12-cup muffin tin.

Cook sausage in a large skillet over medium-high heat until browned and crumbly, 5 to 7 minutes. Drain.

Combine eggs, onion, and chile peppers in a large bowl. Add sausage, salt, and pepper; mix until well combined. Spoon 1/4 cup sausage mixture into each of the prepared muffin cups. Bake in the preheated oven until eggs are set and a toothpick inserted into the center comes out clean, 15 to 20 minutes.

Cheesy Bacon, Sausage, and Egg Hash Brown Skillet

What You Need

6 slices bacon, cut into 1-inch pieces

1 link smoked pineapple-bacon chicken sausage, cut into slices

1 tablespoon canola oil

1 teaspoon butter

2 ½ cups frozen hash brown potatoes, thawed

½ onion, chopped

¾ teaspoon garlic powder, divided

½ teaspoon onion powder

¼ teaspoon salt, or more to taste

¼ teaspoon ground black pepper, or more to taste

1 cup shredded Cheddar cheese

6 large eggs

1 tablespoon milk

Instructions

Preheat the oven to 350 degrees F (175 degrees C).

Place bacon in a 10-inch skillet and cook over medium heat, stirring occasionally, until crisp, about 10 minutes. Use a slotted spoon to remove bacon to a paper towel-lined small bowl. Discard 1/2 of the bacon fat using a spoon.

Cook sausage in remaining bacon fat in the hot skillet until browned on both sides, about 5 minutes. Remove to the bowl with bacon.

Heat canola oil and butter in the same skillet over medium heat. Add hash browns and onion. Stir in 1/2 teaspoon garlic powder, onion powder, salt, and black pepper. Spread hash brown mixture evenly in the skillet; cook, undisturbed, until browned, about 5 minutes. Turn hash browns over and sprinkle with Cheddar cheese.

Whisk together eggs, milk, and remaining 1/4 teaspoon garlic powder in a medium bowl; season with salt and pepper. Pour egg mixture over cheese-covered hash browns in the skillet. Sprinkle the top with bacon and sausage pieces.

Bake in the preheated oven until the top is puffed, cheese is melted, and a knife inserted into the center comes out clean, 10 to 15 minutes.

Peanut Butter and Jelly French Toast Casserole

What You Need

Mini Sandwiches:

14 slices brioche bread

7 tablespoons peanut butter

7 tablespoons jam

Custard:

1 cup 2% milk

3 large eggs

2 tablespoons honey

2 teaspoons vanilla extract

1/4 teaspoon salt

Garnish:

1 tablespoon confectioners sugar, or as needed (optional)

1 tablespoon maple syrup, or as needed (optional)

Instructions

Spray an 8x12-inch to 9x13-inch baking dish with nonstick cooking spray, and set aside.

Spread half of bread slices with peanut butter, and the remainder with jelly, 1 tablespoon each slice. Make 7 sandwiches by combining a peanut butter bread slice with a jelly bread slice.

Brioche is pretty square in shape, so quarter each sandwich, making a total of 28 mini sandwiches. If your bread is a different shape, you may want to consider cutting the mini sandwiches differently. Place the mini sandwiches in rows, cut sides up, in the prepared baking dish, arranging the rows right next to each other.

Make custard: Whisk milk, eggs, honey, vanilla, and salt in a bowl. Drizzle custard over sandwiches, making sure each is well coated. Don't worry if custard pools at the bottom of the dish–the bread will soak it up. Cover casserole with foil, and refrigerate for at least 8 hours or overnight.

Preheat the oven to 350 degrees F (175 degrees C).

Bake casserole in the preheated oven, covered, for 30 minutes. Remove foil, and bake until sandwiches start to crisp and turn golden brown, 20 to 30 minutes more. Sprinkle with confectioners sugar or drizzle with maple syrup.

Overnight Breakfast Bake with Ham, Cheese, and Croissants

What You Need

butter-flavored cooking spray

2 large croissants

½ cup shredded Gruyere cheese

1 cup diced cooked ham

6 large eggs

¾ cup milk

½ cup sour cream

¼ teaspoon salt

¼ teaspoon freshly ground black pepper

1 tablespoon Dijon mustard

2 tablespoons chopped green onions (Optional)

Instructions

Spray an 8x8-inch baking pan with cooking spray.

Cut croissants into 1 inch cubes (about 4 cups, loosely packed) and spread out on the bottom of the prepared pan. Sprinkle evenly with cheese and ham.

Combine eggs, milk, sour cream, Dijon mustard, salt, and pepper in a bowl. Beat the mixture until well blended using a wire whisk or an egg beater.

Pour egg mixture evenly over the top of the croissants, cheese, and ham.

Cover tightly with aluminum foil and place in the refrigerator for 8 hours.

When ready to bake, set the dish out of the refrigerator on the counter, Preheat the oven to 350 degrees F (175 degrees C).

Uncover casserole, place in the center of the preheated oven, and bake until the casserole is set, and a knife inserted into the middle of the casserole comes out clean, 45 to 55 minutes. Cut into serving pieces and garnish with chopped green onions.

Dash's Donair

What You Need

Loaf:

1 teaspoon salt

1 teaspoon ground oregano

1 teaspoon all-purpose flour

½ teaspoon ground black pepper

½ teaspoon Italian seasoning

½ teaspoon garlic powder

½ teaspoon onion powder

¼ teaspoon cayenne pepper

1 pound ground beef

Sauce:

1 (12 fluid ounce) can evaporated milk

¾ cup white sugar

2 teaspoons garlic powder

4 teaspoons white vinegar, or as needed

Instructions

Preheat the oven to 350 degrees F (175 degrees C).

Make loaf: Mix together salt, oregano, flour, black pepper, Italian seasoning, garlic powder, onion powder, and cayenne pepper in a cup or small bowl.

Place ground beef in a large steel mixing bowl on a sturdy surface; use your hands to blend in spice mixture. Pick up meat and throw it down with force about 20 times, kneading it after each throw. This will help meat hold together better when sliced.

Form meat into a loaf; place on a broiler pan or baking sheet.

Bake in the preheated oven for 1 hour and 15 minutes, rotating loaf halfway through to ensure even baking. Serve warm with sauce or allow meat to chill before slicing and reheating. Make sauce: Mix together evaporated milk, sugar, and garlic powder in a medium bowl.

Gradually whisk in white vinegar, 1 teaspoon at a time, until thickened to your desired consistency.

Chilaquiles

What You Need

2 cups oil for frying

30 (6 inch) corn tortillas, torn into strips

¼ cup chopped onion

6 large eggs, lightly beaten

2 teaspoons salt

1 (7.75 ounce) can Mexican-style hot tomato sauce

½ cup water

½ cup shredded Monterey Jack cheese

Instructions

Heat oil in a large, heavy skillet to 350 degrees F (175 degrees C). Fry tortillas and onion in hot oil until crisp and golden brown, stirring frequently. Remove to a paper towel-lined plate to drain. Drain the skillet, leaving only a thin residue of oil.

Place the skillet over medium heat. Return fried tortillas and onion to the skillet and stir in beaten eggs; season with salt. Cook and stir until eggs are firm.

Stir in tomato sauce and water. Reduce heat and simmer until thickened, about 10 minutes. Sprinkle with cheese and continue cooking until cheese is melted.

Chicken Caesar Wrap

What You Need

1 slice bacon

1 cup chopped romaine lettuce

½ cup cooked, shredded chicken

¼ cup croutons

1 tablespoon Caesar's Salad Dressing

1 tablespoon grated Parmesan cheese

1 large flour tortilla

Instructions

Place bacon slice in a large skillet and cook over medium-high heat, turning occasionally, until evenly browned, about 10 minutes. Drain bacon slice on paper towels, cool slightly, and crumble.

Combine bacon, lettuce, shredded chicken, croutons, dressing, and Parmesan cheese for the filling a a bowl. Toss gently to combine and everything is evenly coated with dressing. Adjust dressing amount to your personal preference - for me 1 to 1 1/2 tablespoons is about right.

Warm tortilla in the microwave for about 15 seconds to make it more pliable.

Lay filling What You Need down the center, and roll your wrap up! Enjoy!

Greek Island Chicken Shish Kebabs

What You Need

¼ cup olive oil

¼ cup lemon juice

¼ cup white vinegar

2 cloves garlic, minced

1 teaspoon ground cumin

1 teaspoon dried oregano

½ teaspoon dried thyme

¼ teaspoon salt

¼ teaspoon ground black pepper

2 pounds skinless, boneless chicken breast, cut into 1 1/2-inch pieces

6 wooden skewers

2 large green or red bell peppers, cut into 1-inch pieces

1 large onion, quartered and separated into pieces

12 cherry tomatoes

12 fresh mushrooms

Instructions

Whisk together olive oil, lemon juice, vinegar, garlic, cumin, oregano, thyme, salt, and black pepper in a large glass or ceramic bowl. Add chicken and toss to evenly coat. Cover the bowl with plastic wrap; marinate in the refrigerator for at least 2 hours.

Meanwhile, soak wooden skewers in water for at least 30 minutes before use.

Preheat an outdoor grill for medium-high heat and lightly oil the grate.

Remove chicken from marinade and shake off excess liquid; discard remaining marinade. Alternately thread chicken with bell peppers, onion, tomatoes, and mushrooms onto the skewers.

Cook skewers on the preheated grill, turning frequently, until nicely browned on all sides and chicken is no longer pink in the center, about 10 minutes. An instant-read thermometer inserted into the center should read at least 165 degrees F (74 degrees C).

Briam (Greek Baked Zucchini and Potatoes)

What You Need

2 pounds potatoes, peeled and thinly sliced

4 medium zucchini, thinly sliced

4 small red onions, thinly sliced

6 ripe tomatoes, puréed

½ cup extra-virgin olive oil

2 tablespoons chopped fresh parsley (Optional)

sea salt and freshly ground black pepper to taste

Instructions

Gather all What You Need. Preheat the oven to 400 degrees F (200 degrees C).

Spread potatoes, zucchini, and red onions in an extra-large baking dish (9x13-inch or larger, or 2 baking dishes).

Cover with puréed tomatoes, olive oil, and parsley; season liberally with sea salt and pepper. Toss until vegetables are evenly coated.

Bake in the preheated oven for 1 hour. Stir gently, then continue baking until vegetables are tender and moisture has evaporated, about 30 minutes more.

Zucchini Artichoke Summer Salad

What You Need

2 skinless, boneless chicken breast halves

salt and ground black pepper to taste

6 tablespoons olive oil, divided

4 zucchini, cut into 1 1/2-inch sticks

1 (15 ounce) can garbanzo beans, drained and rinsed

1 (6 ounce) can black olives, drained and sliced

1 (14 ounce) can artichoke hearts, drained and chopped

½ cup grated Parmesan cheese

Instructions

Season both sides of chicken breasts with salt and black pepper.

Heat 2 tablespoons olive oil in a skillet over medium heat; cook chicken breasts in the hot oil until they are no longer pink in the center and juices run clear, 5 to 10 minutes per side. An instant-read thermometer inserted into the thickest part of a breast should read at least 165 degrees F (74 degrees C). Cut chicken into 1/2-inch cubes and transfer to a large bowl.

Heat remaining 4 tablespoons olive oil in the same skillet over medium heat; cook and stir zucchini in the hot oil until slightly tender, about 5 minutes. Season with salt and black pepper. Transfer zucchini to a paper towel-lined plate to drain.

Mix zucchini, garbanzo beans, olives, artichoke hearts, and Parmesan cheese with chicken; toss to combine. Chill in refrigerator before serving, about 1 hour.

Avocado and Tuna Tapas

What You Need

1 (12 ounce) can solid white tuna packed in water, drained

1 tablespoon mayonnaise

3 green onions, thinly sliced, plus additional for garnish

½ red bell pepper, chopped

1 dash balsamic vinegar

black pepper to taste

1 pinch garlic salt, or to taste

2 ripe avocados, halved and pitted

Instructions

Stir together tuna, mayonnaise, green onions, red pepper, and balsamic vinegar in a bowl. Season with pepper and garlic salt, then pack the avocado halves with the tuna mixture.

Garnish with reserved green onions and a dash of black pepper before serving.

Greek Salad

What You Need

2 large English cucumbers

1 pinch kosher salt

2 cups cherry tomatoes

¼ red onion

½ red bell pepper

½ cup pitted Kalamata olives

½ cup pitted green olives

2 tablespoons minced fresh oregano

salt and freshly ground black pepper to taste

1 pinch cayenne pepper, or to taste

¼ cup red wine vinegar, or to taste

⅓ cup olive oil, or to taste

1 (4 ounce) package feta cheese, diced, divided

1 teaspoon minced fresh oregano, or to taste

Instructions

Peel off a few strips of cucumber skin using a channel knife, creating a striped pattern. Cut cucumbers in half crosswise. Cut each half into quarters before cutting into 1/4- to 1/2-inch slices. Place into a colander; toss with some kosher salt and let sit for 10 to 15 minutes.

Meanwhile, cut cherry tomatoes in half. Rinse cucumbers; drain thoroughly for 10 to 15 minutes more.

While cucumbers are draining, slice onion thinly. Cut bell pepper into strips. Turn knife diagonally and cut strips into diamond-shaped pieces. Slice Kalamata and green olives.

Combine cucumbers, tomatoes, onion, bell pepper, olives, and 2 tablespoons oregano in a bowl. Season with salt, black pepper, and cayenne. Sprinkle in vinegar and toss thoroughly. Drizzle in olive oil. Add about 2/3 of the feta cheese and toss again. Cover with plastic wrap and refrigerate for 30 to 60 minutes.

Give the salad another mix. Taste and season as desired. Scatter remaining feta cheese on top and garnish with remaining oregano.

KIDNEY-FRIENDLY LUNCH IDEAS

Scallops Provencale

What You Need

2 tablespoons butter

1 pound sea scallops, rinsed and drained

1 small onion, finely chopped

½ pound mushrooms, thinly sliced

1 clove garlic, minced

2 medium tomatoes, peeled and chopped

¼ cup dry white wine (Optional)

2 tablespoons ketchup

½ teaspoon salt

½ teaspoon chopped dried tarragon

¼ teaspoon dried rosemary

1 pinch white pepper

¼ pound frozen, small, cooked shrimp

2 teaspoons white wine vinegar

chopped fresh parsley, for garnish

Instructions

Heat butter in a large skillet over medium-high heat. Without crowding, lightly brown scallops in batches. Remove scallops to individual casseroles or lightly buttered baking shells.

Stir onion and mushrooms into the skillet, and cook until the onion is soft and begins to brown. Stir in garlic, tomatoes, wine, ketchup, salt, tarragon, rosemary, and white pepper. Bring to a boil; cover, reduce heat to low, and simmer 15 minutes. Uncover, and cook until thick, about 3 minutes. Mix in shrimp and vinegar.

Preheat oven to 400 degrees F (200 degrees C). Spoon sauce evenly over scallops.

Bake in a preheated oven until sauce bubbles and begins to brown at the edges, about 10 minutes. Sprinkle parsley over tops, and serve.

Marinated Green Beans with Olives, Tomatoes, and Feta

What You Need

2 pounds fresh green beans, trimmed

¼ cup olive oil

2 cloves garlic, minced

1 cup kalamata olives, pitted and sliced

2 tomatoes, seeded and chopped

2 tablespoons red wine vinegar

1 tablespoon chopped fresh oregano

½ teaspoon salt

¼ teaspoon ground black pepper

1 (8 ounce) package crumbled feta

1 bunch fresh oregano sprigs

Instructions

Bring a large pot of salted water to a boil over medium heat. Add green beans; cook until slightly tender, but still crisp, 8 to 10 minutes. Immediately drain green beans and plunge them into ice water to stop cooking further.

Drain beans and place them in a shallow serving dish.

Heat olive oil in a skillet over medium heat. Cook garlic in oil for about 30 seconds. Remove the skillet from heat. Stir in olives, tomatoes, vinegar, oregano, salt, and pepper.

Pour mixture over green beans; toss together until beans are evenly coated. Sprinkle feta cheese on top and garnish with oregano sprigs. Chill at least 3 hours before serving.

Pan-Seared Scallops with Pepper and Onions in Anchovy Oil

What You Need

⅓ cup extra virgin olive oil

1 (2 ounce) can anchovy fillets, minced

1 pound large sea scallops

1 large red bell pepper, coarsely chopped

1 large orange bell pepper, coarsely chopped

1 red onion, coarsely chopped

2 cloves garlic, thinly sliced

1 teaspoon minced lime zest

1 ½ teaspoons minced lemon zest

1 pinch kosher salt and pepper to taste

8 sprigs fresh parsley, for garnish

Instructions

Heat the olive oil and minced anchovies in a large skillet over medium-high heat, stirring as the oil heats to dissolve the anchovies. Once the anchovies are sizzling, add the sea scallops, and cook without moving the scallops for 2 minutes.

Meanwhile, toss red bell pepper, orange bell pepper, red onion, garlic, lime zest, and lemon zest in a bowl; season with salt and pepper. Sprinkle pepper mixture onto the scallops and continue cooking until scallops have browned, about 2 minutes more. Turn scallops, stir the pepper mixture, and continue cooking until the scallops have browned on the other side, 4 to 5 minutes. Garnish with parsley sprigs to serve.

Braised Chicken and Artichoke Hearts with Lemon, Cherry Peppers and Thyme

What You Need

1 tablespoon olive oil

4 chicken leg quarters

1 yellow onion, chopped

4 cloves garlic, chopped

1 tablespoon fresh ground black pepper

1 teaspoon salt

½ teaspoon red pepper flakes

1 quart chicken stock or low-sodium broth

10 canned artichoke hearts, drained and halved

2 cups cherry peppers

2 lemons, juiced

8 sprigs fresh thyme

1 (16 ounce) can butter beans, drained

Instructions

Preheat the oven to 375 degrees F (190 degrees C).

Coat bottom of a Dutch oven with olive oil and place over high-heat. Sear chicken until browned, about 5 minutes per side. Transfer to a warm plate.

Stir onion, garlic, black pepper, salt, and red pepper flakes into the Dutch oven; cook and stir for 1 minute. Stir in chicken broth and return to a simmer. Remove from heat.

Return chicken to the Dutch oven. Stir in artichoke hearts, cherry peppers, lemon juice, and thyme.

Cover Dutch oven and place in the preheated oven. Cook until chicken is tender, about 1 hour.

Remove Dutch oven and transfer chicken to a warm plate.

Stir beans into the Dutch oven with broth and artichoke mixture.

Serve each chicken leg quarter in a bowl. Pour a ladle-full of artichoke, bean, and broth mixture over each.

Insalata Caprese

What You Need

4 large ripe tomatoes, sliced 1/4 inch thick

1 pound fresh mozzarella cheese, sliced 1/4 inch thick

⅓ cup fresh basil leaves

3 tablespoons extra virgin olive oil

fine sea salt and freshly ground black pepper to taste

Instructions

Alternate and overlap tomato slices, mozzarella cheese slices, and basil leaves on a large platter. Drizzle with olive oil. Season with sea salt and pepper.

Cucumber Sandwiches

What You Need

1 cucumber, peeled and thinly sliced

1 (8 ounce) package cream cheese, softened

¼ cup mayonnaise

¼ teaspoon garlic powder

¼ teaspoon onion salt

1 dash Worcestershire sauce

1 (1 pound) loaf sliced bread, crusts removed

1 pinch lemon pepper (Optional)

Instructions

Place cucumber slices between 2 paper towels set in a colander. Allow liquid to drain, about 10 minutes.

Mix cream cheese, mayonnaise, garlic powder, onion salt, and Worcestershire sauce in a bowl until smooth.

Spread cream cheese mixture evenly on one side of each bread slice.

Divide cucumber slices over half of the bread slices; sprinkle lemon pepper on cucumber.

Stack the other half of the bread slices spread-side down over cucumber to make sandwiches; slice into triangles.

Tips

To serve as a party appetizer, cut bread slices into rounds with a cookie cutter. Spread with cream cheese mixture and top each with a cucumber slice. Yields approximately 48 rounds.

To make these the night before, cover with slightly damp paper towels, then cover with foil; store in the fridge.

Spiced Sweet Roasted Red Pepper Hummus

What You Need

1 (15 ounce) can garbanzo beans, drained

1 (4 ounce) jar roasted red peppers

3 tablespoons lemon juice

1 ½ tablespoons tahini

1 clove garlic, minced

½ teaspoon ground cumin

½ teaspoon cayenne pepper

¼ teaspoon salt

1 tablespoon chopped fresh parsley

Instructions

In an electric blender or food processor, purée garbanzo beans, red peppers, lemon juice, tahini, garlic, cumin, cayenne, and salt. Use long pulses to process until mixture is fairly smooth and slightly fluffy, scraping down the sides in between pulses. Transfer to a serving bowl and refrigerate for at least 1 hour or up to 3 days.

Return to room temperature and sprinkle with chopped parsley before serving.

Lemon Chicken Piccata

What You Need

3 large skinless, boneless chicken breast halves - cut into 1/2-inch medallions

salt and pepper to taste

½ cup all-purpose flour

2 tablespoons vegetable oil, or as needed

1 clove garlic, minced

1 cup low sodium chicken broth

½ lemon, thinly sliced

¼ cup fresh lemon juice

2 tablespoons capers, drained and rinsed

3 tablespoons butter

2 tablespoons minced Italian (flat-leaf) parsley

Instructions

Preheat oven to 200 degrees F (95 degrees C). Place a serving platter into the oven to warm.

Season the chicken breast pieces with salt and pepper and dredge them in flour. Shake off excess flour. Heat the vegetable oil in a skillet; pan-fry the chicken pieces until golden brown on both sides, about 3 minutes per side. Work in batches and do not crowd skillet, adding oil as needed . Place the chicken pieces onto the warmed platter in the oven. When finished with all the chicken, drain most of the oil from the skillet, leaving a thin coating on the surface of the pan.

Cook and stir the minced garlic in the skillet until fragrant, about 20 seconds. Pour in the chicken broth. Scrape and dissolve any brown bits from the bottom of the skillet. Stir in the lemon slices and bring the mixture to a boil. Let cook, stirring occasionally, until the sauce reduces to about 2/3 cup, 5 to 8 minutes. Add the lemon juice and capers; simmer until the sauce is reduced and slightly thickened, about 5 minutes more. Drop the butter into the skillet and swirl it into the sauce by tilting the skillet until the butter is melted and incorporated. Add the parsley; remove from heat and set aside.

Arrange the chicken medallions on serving plates and spoon sauce over each portion to serve.

Broiled Spanish Mackerel

What You Need

6 (3 ounce) fillets Spanish mackerel fillets

¼ cup olive oil

½ teaspoon paprika

salt and ground black pepper to taste

12 slices lemon

Instructions

Preheat the oven's broiler and set the oven rack about 6 inches from the heat source. Lightly grease a baking dish.

Rub both sides of each mackerel fillet with olive oil and place with the skin side down into the prepared baking dish. Season each fillet with the paprika, salt, and pepper. Top each fillet with two lemon slices.

Bake the fillets under the broiler until the fish just begins to flake, 5 to 7 minutes. Serve immediately.

Fried Soft-Shell Crab

What You Need

4 soft-shell crabs

1 quart oil for frying, or as needed

½ cup milk

1 large egg

1 cup all-purpose flour

salt and pepper to taste

Instructions

Lift one pointed side of the top shell of one crab; pull out and discard the gills. Lower the shell and repeat on the other side. Remove the tail flap on the bottom side by twisting and pulling. Use a pair of scissors to cut behind the eyes and remove the face. Repeat to clean remaining crabs. Rinse cleaned crabs thoroughly with cold water, then dry on paper towels.

Heat oil in a deep fryer to 365 degrees F (180 degrees C).

Whisk together milk and egg in a shallow bowl. Combine flour, salt, and pepper in another shallow bowl. Lightly salt each crab. Dredge in flour; shake off excess. Dip into beaten egg. Lift up so excess egg drips back into the bowl. Press into flour to coat both sides.

Working in batches if necessary, carefully lower crabs into the hot oil and fry until golden brown on one side, 1 to 2 minutes. Carefully turn and cook until golden brown on the other side, 1 to 2 minutes more. Drain on paper towels.

Pan-Seared Salmon

What You Need

4 (6 ounce) fillets salmon

2 tablespoons olive oil

2 tablespoons capers

⅛ teaspoon salt

⅛ teaspoon ground black pepper

4 slices lemon

Instructions

Preheat a large heavy skillet over medium heat for 3 minutes.

Coat salmon fillets with olive oil; place skin-side down in the preheated skillet and increase heat to high.

Sprinkle with capers, salt, and pepper; cook for 3 minutes on one side. Turn salmon fillets over; continue to cook until salmon flakes easily with a fork, about 5 minutes.

Transfer salmon to individual plates and garnish with lemon slices.

Capers and Halibut

What You Need

1 tablespoon olive oil

2 (8 ounce) steaks halibut

½ cup white wine

¼ cup butter

1 teaspoon chopped garlic

3 tablespoons capers, with liquid

salt and pepper to taste

Instructions

Heat oil in a large skillet over medium-high heat. Add halibut steaks and sear until nicely browned, 2 to 3 minutes per side. Transfer to a plate.

Pour wine into the pan and bring to a boil while scraping the browned bits of food off the bottom of the pan with a wooden spoon. Cook until wine is almost completely gone, then stir in garlic, butter, and capers. Season with salt and pepper, then simmer for about 1 minute to blend the flavors.

Return halibut steaks to the pan. Spoon sauce over steaks to coat; cook until fish flakes easily with a fork, 2 to 3 more minutes.

To serve, cut steaks in half and pour pan sauce over top.

Spanish Moroccan Fish

What You Need

1 tablespoon vegetable oil

1 onion, chopped

1 clove garlic, finely chopped

1 (15 ounce) can garbanzo beans, drained and rinsed

2 red bell peppers, seeded and sliced into strips

1 large carrot, thinly sliced

3 tomatoes, chopped

4 olives, chopped

¼ cup chopped fresh parsley

¼ cup ground cumin

3 tablespoons paprika

2 tablespoons chicken bouillon granules

1 teaspoon cayenne pepper

salt, to taste

5 pounds tilapia fillets

Instructions

Heat vegetable oil in a skillet over medium heat. Stir in onion and garlic; cook and stir until onion has softened and turned translucent, about 5 minutes. Add garbanzo beans, bell peppers, carrots, tomatoes, and olives; continue to cook until peppers are slightly tender, about 5 minutes more.

Sprinkle parsley, cumin, paprika, chicken bouillon, and cayenne over vegetables. Season with salt. Stir to incorporate. Place tilapia on top of vegetables and add enough water to cover vegetables. Reduce heat to low, cover, and cook until fish flakes easily with a fork and juices run clear, about 40 minutes.

Nicoise-Style Tuna Salad With White Beans & Olives

What You Need

¾ pound green beans, trimmed and snapped in half

1 (12 ounce) can solid white albacore tuna, drained

1 (16 ounce) can Great Northern beans, drained and rinsed

1 (2.25 ounce) can sliced black olives, drained

¼ medium red onion, thinly sliced

1 teaspoon dried oregano

6 tablespoons extra-virgin olive oil

3 tablespoons lemon juice

½ teaspoon finely grated lemon zest

Salt and ground black pepper, to taste

4 large hard-cooked eggs, peeled and quartered

Instructions

Place green beans, 1/3 cup water and a large pinch of salt in a medium skillet. Cover, turn heat on high, and bring water to boil. Once beans start to steam, set timer and cook until tender-crisp, about 5 minutes. (Because the beans cook in such a small amount of water, make sure not to let the skillet run dry.) Immediately dump them onto a lipped cookie sheet lined with paper towels to cool.

Mix tuna, white beans, olives and onion in a medium bowl. Whisk together oregano, oil, lemon juice and zest in a medium bowl, then pour over the salad and gently stir to combine. Adjust seasonings to taste. Arrange a portion of green beans, tuna-bean salad and eggs on each of 4 plates.

Cucumber Gazpacho

What You Need

2 large English cucumbers

3 cups chopped honeydew melon

1 cup cubed crustless day-old white bread

¼ cup olive oil, plus extra for drizzling

1 tablespoon sherry vinegar

2 ¼ teaspoons kosher salt, plus more to taste

¼ cup crumbled feta cheese

2 tablespoons chopped fresh mint

2 teaspoons honey

Instructions

Thinly slice one of the cucumbers to equal 1/3 cup. Transfer cucumber slices to a small bowl; cover and chill until ready to use.

Coarsely chop remaining cucumbers and transfer to a blender. Add honeydew, bread cubes, 1/4 cup oil, vinegar, and 2 1/4 teaspoons kosher salt. Process on low speed, gradually increasing speed to high, until cucumber mixture is very smooth and creamy, about 90 seconds.

Pour gazpacho into a medium bowl. Cover and chill until cold, about 1 hour.

Right before serving, toss together reserved cucumber slices, feta cheese, mint, honey, and a pinch of salt in a small bowl.

Stir and ladle gazpacho into 4 shallow bowls. Top evenly with cucumber-feta mixture and drizzle with olive oil.

KIDNEY-SUPPORTIVE DINNER IDEAS

Garlic Escargots

What You Need

1 (7 ounce) can escargots, drained

6 tablespoons butter

1 clove garlic, minced

20 mushrooms, stems removed

⅓ cup white wine

⅓ cup cream

1 tablespoon all-purpose flour

¼ teaspoon dried tarragon

1 pinch freshly ground black pepper, or to taste

¼ cup grated Parmesan cheese

Instructions

Place escargots in a small bowl and cover with cold water. Let sit for 5 minutes to remove any canned flavor they may have.

Preheat the oven to 350 degrees F (175 degrees C). Lightly grease an 8x8-inch baking dish.

Drain escargots and pat dry with a paper towel.

Melt butter with garlic in a large skillet over medium-high heat. Add escargots and mushroom caps; cook and stir until mushroom caps begin to soften, about 5 minutes.

Whisk together wine, cream, flour, tarragon, and pepper in a small bowl until well combined. Pour into the skillet and bring to a boil. Cook, stirring occasionally, until sauce thickens, about 10 minutes. Remove from the heat.

Place mushroom caps into the prepared baking dish, with the tops facing down. Spoon an escargot into each mushroom cap. Pour sauce from the skillet over mushroom caps, then sprinkle grated Parmesan cheese over top.

Bake in the preheated oven until cheese has turned golden brown, 10 to 15 minutes.

Oven Roasted Red Potatoes and Asparagus

What You Need

1 ½ pounds red potatoes, cut into chunks

2 tablespoons extra-virgin olive oil, divided

8 cloves garlic, thinly sliced

4 teaspoons dried rosemary

4 teaspoons dried thyme

2 teaspoons kosher salt, divided

1 bunch fresh asparagus, trimmed and cut into 1 inch pieces

ground black pepper to taste

Instructions

Preheat the oven to 425 degrees F (220 degrees C).

Toss potatoes with 1 tablespoon oil, garlic, rosemary, thyme, and 1 teaspoon salt in a large baking dish. Cover with aluminum foil.

Bake in the preheated oven for 20 minutes.

Mix in asparagus, remaining 1 tablespoon oil, and remaining 1 teaspoon salt. Cover and continue to cook until potatoes are tender, about 15 minutes.

Increase oven temperature to 450 degrees F (230 degrees C). Remove foil and cook until potatoes are lightly browned, 5 to 10 more minutes. Season with pepper.

Dutch Apple Pie with Oatmeal Streusel

What You Need

Apple Pie:

5 cups apples - peeled, cored and sliced

⅔ cup white sugar

2 tablespoons all-purpose flour

½ teaspoon ground cinnamon

¼ teaspoon ground nutmeg

¼ teaspoon ground allspice

1 (9 inch) frozen pie crust

2 tablespoons butter

aluminum foil

Streusel Topping:

¾ cup all-purpose flour

¾ cup rolled oats

½ cup packed brown sugar

1 teaspoon lemon zest

½ teaspoon ground cinnamon

½ cup butter

Instructions

Preheat the oven to 425 degrees F (220 degrees C).

Make the apple pie: Place apple slices in a large bowl. Mix white sugar, flour, cinnamon, nutmeg, and allspice together in a separate bowl until combined; sprinkle over apples and toss until evenly coated.

Remove pie shell from freezer; pour apple mixture into pie shell and dot with butter. Lay a sheet of aluminum foil lightly on top of filling, but do not seal.

Bake pie in the preheated oven for 10 minutes. Meanwhile, make the streusel topping: Mix flour, oats, brown sugar, lemon zest, and cinnamon in a medium bowl until combined.

Cut in butter until mixture is crumbly. Remove pie from oven and sprinkle streusel on top. Reduce heat to 375 degrees F (190 degrees C). Return pie to oven and bake until streusel is browned and apples are tender, 30 to 35 minutes more. Cover loosely with aluminum foil to prevent excess browning.

Baked Mac and Cheese with Sour Cream and Cottage Cheese

What You Need

cooking spray

1 (16 ounce) package elbow macaroni

2 (8 ounce) packages mild Cheddar cheese, shredded, divided

1 (8 ounce) package sharp Cheddar cheese, shredded

¾ cup sour cream

¾ cup cottage cheese

1 large egg

salt and ground black pepper to taste

Instructions

Preheat the oven to 350 degrees F (175 degrees C). Spray a 9x13-inch baking dish with cooking spray.

Bring a large pot of lightly salted water to a boil. Cook elbow macaroni in the boiling water, stirring occasionally, until cooked through but firm to the bite, 8 minutes; drain.

Reserve 1/2 cup shredded mild Cheddar cheese; set aside.

Mix together remaining mild Cheddar cheese, sharp Cheddar cheese, sour cream, cottage cheese, and egg in a bowl; season with salt and pepper. Stir cooked macaroni into cheese mixture. Pour macaroni mixture into the prepared baking dish; sprinkle with reserved 1/2 cup mild Cheddar cheese.

Bake in the preheated oven until cheese is melted and bubbling, about 40 minutes. Let cool for 10 minutes before serving.

Baked Feta Cheese and Tomatoes

What You Need

1 (7 ounce) block Greek feta cheese

1 tablespoon honey

drizzle of olive oil

2 cups halved cherry or grape tomatoes

1/3 cup halved Kalamata olives

1/3 cup thinly sliced red onion

2 tablespoons olive oil

1 clove garlic, minced

1 teaspoon dried oregano

salt and freshly ground black pepper to taste

chopped fresh basil for garnish (optional)

Instructions

Preheat the oven to 400 degrees F (200 degrees C).

Place the feta cheese in the center of a baking dish. Spread with honey and drizzle with olive oil.

In a small bowl, combine tomatoes, olives, red onion, olive oil, and garlic. Sprinkle with oregano, season with salt and pepper, and toss. Arrange the tomato mixture around the feta cheese.

Bake in the preheated oven until cheese is soft and tomato mixture is bubbly, 20 to 30 minutes. If you want more color, briefly place under the broiler.

Garnish with fresh basil, if desired, and serve warm.

Tuna Casserole

What You Need

3 cups cooked macaroni

1 (5 ounce) can tuna, drained

1 (10.5 ounce) can condensed cream of chicken soup

1 cup shredded Cheddar cheese

1 ½ cups French fried onions

Instructions

Preheat the oven to 350 degrees F (175 degrees C).

Combine cooked macaroni, tuna, and condensed soup together in a 9x13-inch baking dish; sprinkle with cheese.

Bake in the preheated oven until bubbly, about 25 minutes. Sprinkle with fried onions; bake 5 minutes more.

Balsamic Grilled Zucchini

What You Need

2 zucchinis, quartered lengthwise

2 teaspoons olive oil

1 teaspoon Italian seasoning

½ teaspoon garlic powder

1 pinch salt

2 tablespoons balsamic vinegar

Instructions

Gather all What You Need.

Preheat an outdoor grill for medium-low heat and lightly oil the grate.

Brush zucchini with olive oil. Sprinkle Italian seasoning, garlic powder, and salt over zucchini.

Cook on the preheated grill until beginning to brown, 3 to 4 minutes per side. Brush balsamic vinegar over zucchini and continue cooking 1 minute more.

Serve immediately.

Italian Rice Balls

What You Need

2 large eggs

⅓ cup grated Parmesan cheese

1 tablespoon dried parsley

2 teaspoons salt, divided

¼ teaspoon freshly ground black pepper

1 quart water

1 cup uncooked white rice

1 ½ cups dried bread crumbs

2 cups olive oil, or as needed

Instructions

Whisk together eggs, cheese, parsley, 1 teaspoon salt, and pepper in a medium bowl until combined. Cover the bowl and place in the refrigerator while you prepare rice.

Pour water and remaining 1 teaspoon salt into a large saucepan; bring to a boil. Stir in rice and reduce heat to low. Cook rice, stirring frequently, until water is almost completely absorbed. Remove from heat and slowly pour in egg mixture, stirring rapidly to prevent egg from scrambling. Allow rice mixture to cool at room temperature for 1 hour.

Pour bread crumbs into a pile on one end of a cutting board. Dampen hands and roll rice mixture into 1-inch balls, then coat each one with bread crumbs.

Heat 1 inch oil in a deep saucepan to 350 degrees F (175 degrees C).

Working in batches, fry rice balls in hot oil, turning as needed to ensure even browning. Drain on paper towels and serve warm.

Mushroom Rice

What You Need

2 teaspoons butter

6 mushrooms, coarsely chopped

1 green onion, finely chopped

1 clove garlic, minced

2 cups chicken broth

1 cup uncooked white rice

½ teaspoon chopped fresh parsley

salt and pepper to taste

Instructions

Melt butter in a saucepan over medium heat. Cook mushrooms, green onion, and garlic in butter until mushrooms are cooked and liquid has evaporated, about 5 minutes.

Stir in chicken broth and rice. Season with parsley, salt, and pepper. Bring to a boil, then reduce heat. Cover and simmer until liquid is absorbed, about 20 minutes.

Grilled Pattypan Squash With Garlic Butter

What You Need

4 tablespoons unsalted butter, softened

1 tablespoon finely chopped flat-leaf parsley

1 clove garlic, finely minced

1 1/4 teaspoons kosher salt, divided

3/4 teaspoon freshly ground black pepper, divided

1 1/2 pounds pattypan squash

1 tablespoon olive oil

Instructions

Preheat grill or grill pan to medium-high (400 to 450 degrees F; 200 to 230 degrees C). Stir together butter, parsley, garlic, and 1/4 teaspoon each of the salt and pepper in a small bowl. Set aside.

For larger pieces of pattypan squash, trim stem ends and cut into quarters or wedges. For smaller squash, cut in half.

Toss together cut squash, olive oil, and remaining 1 teaspoon salt and 1/2 teaspoon pepper. Place pieces of squash on oiled grates, and grill, undisturbed, until they release easily from the grill with distinct grill marks, 3 to 5 minutes. Flip squash, and continue to cook until tender and cooked on each side, about 5 minutes more. Place in a shallow dish for serving.

Top hot grilled squash with garlic butter, and serve immediately.

Crisp Pickled Green Beans

What You Need

2 ½ cups distilled white vinegar

2 cups water

¼ cup salt

1 clove garlic, peeled

2 ½ pounds fresh green beans

6 large sprigs dill

¾ teaspoon red pepper flakes (Optional)

Instructions

Inspect six 1/2-pint jars for cracks and rings for rust, discarding any defective ones. Immerse in simmering water. Wash new, unused lids and rings in warm soapy water.

While the jars are bring sterilized, stir together vinegar, water, and salt in a large saucepan. Add garlic and bring to a rolling boil over high heat.

Trim green beans to 1/4-inch shorter than the jars.

Remove jars from simmering water. Place 1 sprig of dill and 1/8 teaspoon red pepper flakes in each jar. Pack in green beans standing on end.

Ladle boiling brine (leave out garlic) into the jars, filling within 1/4-inch of the tops. Seal jars with lids and rings.

Place a rack in the bottom of a large stockpot and fill halfway with water. Bring to a boil and lower jars 2 inches apart into the boiling water using a holder. Pour in more boiling water to cover jars by at least 1 inch. Bring to a simmer (do not boil), cover, and process for 10 minutes. Remove jars from the stockpot and cool to room temperature, 8 to 12 hours. Test jars for a good seal by pressing on the center of the lid — it should not move.

Let green beans ferment for 2 to 3 weeks in a cool, dark space before eating.

Sausage Stuffed Jalapeños

What You Need

1 pound ground pork sausage

1 (8 ounce) package cream cheese, softened

1 cup shredded Parmesan cheese

1 pound large fresh jalapeno peppers, halved lengthwise and seeded

1 (8 ounce) bottle Ranch dressing (Optional)

Instructions

Gather all What You Need.

Preheat the oven to 425 degrees F (220 degrees C).

Place sausage in a skillet over medium heat. Cook and stir until evenly brown; drain.

Mix sausage, cream cheese, and Parmesan cheese together in a large bowl.

Spoon about 1 tablespoon of sausage mixture into each jalapeño half; arrange stuffed halves in baking dishes.

Bake in the preheated oven until bubbly and lightly browned, about 20 minutes. Serve with ranch dressing.

Stuffed Pork Chops

What You Need

2 tablespoons vegetable oil

4 thick cut pork chops

3 cups day-old bread cubes

¼ cup butter, melted

¼ cup chicken broth

2 tablespoons chopped celery

2 tablespoons chopped onion

¼ teaspoon poultry seasoning

1 (10.5 ounce) can condensed cream of mushroom soup

⅓ cup water

Instructions

Preheat the oven to 350 degrees F (175 degrees C).

Heat oil in a large skillet over medium heat. Add pork chops and cook until browned, 4 to 6 minutes per side; transfer to a baking dish.

Toss bread cubes, melted butter, chicken broth, celery, onion, and poultry seasoning together in a medium bowl. Spoon heaping mounds of the stuffing mixture onto the pork chops.

Combine condensed soup with water; pour over the stuffing and pork chops. Cover the baking dish with aluminum foil.

Bake in preheated oven for 30 minutes. Remove foil and continue baking for 10 minutes longer or until juices run clear. A meat thermometer inserted into the center of a pork chop should read 145 degrees F (63 degrees C).

'Chinese Buffet' Green Beans

What You Need

1 tablespoon oil, peanut or sesame

2 cloves garlic, thinly sliced

1 pound fresh green beans, trimmed

2 tablespoons oyster sauce

1 tablespoon white sugar

2 teaspoons soy sauce

Instructions

Heat oil in a wok or large skillet over medium-high heat. Stir in garlic; cook until edges begin to brown, about 20 seconds. Add green beans; cook and stir until they begin to soften, about 5 minutes.

Stir in oyster sauce, sugar, and soy sauce. Cook and stir until beans have attained the desired degree of tenderness, 2 to 4 minutes.

Asparagus Wrapped in Crisp Prosciutto

What You Need

1 tablespoon olive oil

16 spears fresh asparagus, trimmed

16 slices prosciutto

Instructions

Preheat the oven to 450 degrees F (220 degrees C). Line a baking sheet with aluminum foil, and coat with olive oil.

Wrap one slice of prosciutto around each asparagus spear, starting at the bottom, and spiraling up to the tip. Place the wrapped spears on the prepared baking sheet.

Bake in the preheated oven for 5 minutes. Remove, and shake the pan back and forth to roll the spears over. Return to the oven until asparagus is tender and prosciutto is crisp, another 5 minutes. Serve immediately.

KIDNEY-FRIENDLY SOUP RECIPES

Chilled Corn Soup

What You Need

1 tablespoon olive oil

1 clove garlic, smashed and peeled

2 green onions, white and tender green parts separated and chopped

¾ teaspoon ground coriander

¾ teaspoon cumin

¾ teaspoon chipotle chile powder

3 cups fresh corn kernels (from fresh ears of corn or frozen corn, thawed)

1 cup buttermilk

½ cup water

½ teaspoon salt

¼ cup chopped cilantro (Optional)

Instructions

Heat oil in a skillet over medium-low heat. Cook garlic, white parts of onions, coriander, cumin, and chile powder, stirring, until garlic and onions are tender, about 3 minutes. Add corn and cook, stirring occasionally, until tender, about 2 minutes.

Transfer mixture to a blender. Add buttermilk, water, and salt and puree until smooth. Strain through a fine-mesh sieve, pressing on solids to extract as much liquid as possible. Discard solids. Chill at least 1 hour.

Serve chilled, garnished with green parts of onions and cilantro (if using).

Roasted Carrot and Tahini Soup

What You Need

1 ½ pounds carrots, peeled and cut 1-inch pieces

1 small yellow onion, cut into 1-inch pieces

3 cloves garlic, peeled

2 tablespoons olive oil

½ teaspoon salt

¼ teaspoon ground black pepper

4 cups vegetable broth

⅓ cup tahini

½ teaspoon curry powder

½ teaspoon ground coriander

¼ teaspoon ground ginger

⅛ teaspoon ground turmeric

⅛ teaspoon ground cardamom

⅓ cup heavy cream

salt and ground black pepper to taste

Instructions

Preheat the oven to 400 degrees F (200 degrees C). Line a large baking sheet with aluminum foil.

Combine carrots, onion, and garlic in a large bowl. Drizzle with olive oil and season with salt and pepper. Toss to coat. Spread vegetables evenly on the baking sheet.

Roast in the preheated oven until lightly browned and soft, about 25 minutes.

Combine 2 cups vegetable broth with 1/2 of the cooked vegetables in a blender jar. Puree until smooth and pour into a large saucepan over medium heat. Puree remaining broth and vegetables with tahini; pour into the saucepan.

Add curry powder, coriander, ginger, turmeric, and cardamom to the vegetable puree. Stir until warm. Stir in heavy cream and remove from heat. Season with salt and pepper. Ladle soup into bowls.

Bone Broth

What You Need

7 pounds beef bones, such as oxtail, short rib, knuckle, and shank

6 quarts water

2 tablespoons red wine vinegar

3 onions, coarsely chopped

3 carrots, coarsely chopped

3 stalks celery, coarsely chopped

1 head garlic, cloves separated and peeled

2 cups parsley leaves

12 sprigs fresh thyme

2 bay leaves

1 tablespoon whole black peppercorns

⅓ cup dried mushrooms, such as porcini

Instructions

Preheat oven to 400 degrees F (200 degrees C). Arrange bones on 2 rimmed baking sheets and roast, turning occasionally, until well browned, about 45 minutes. Transfer bones to a 12-quart stockpot. Pour off fat from baking sheets, reserving 1 tablespoon. Add water and vinegar to pot and bring to a boil. Reduce heat and gently simmer, skimming off foam occasionally, 1 1/2 hours.

Meanwhile, arrange onions, carrots, celery, and garlic on baking sheet (from roasting bones) and drizzle with reserved fat. Roast vegetables, tossing occasionally, until softened, about 40 minutes.

Add vegetables to pot with bones, then stir in parsley, thyme, bay leaves, peppercorns, and mushrooms. Keep heat low enough that liquid barely simmers, and cook 12 hours (overnight). Strain soup through a fine-mesh sieve and discard solids. Skim any remaining foam and taste broth. To intensify flavor, transfer soup to a clean pot and boil to desired concentration.

Spinach Artichoke Soup

What You Need

1 (32 ounce) container chicken broth

1 ½ cups shredded cooked chicken

½ cup chopped onion

2 large cloves garlic, chopped

1 (10 ounce) package frozen chopped spinach, thawed

½ (14 ounce) can quartered artichoke hearts, drained and chopped

½ (8 ounce) package reduced-fat cream cheese

Instructions

Combine chicken broth, chicken, onion, and garlic in a large pot over medium heat. Bring to a boil; reduce heat and simmer until onion is tender, about 10 minutes.

Stir spinach and artichoke hearts into the pot. Bring broth back to a simmer. Drop in cream cheese in large spoonfuls, stirring continuously until melted, about 5 minutes.

Roasted Apple and Parsnip Soup

What You Need

2 pounds parsnips, peeled and cut into 1/2-inch slices

2 green apples - peeled, cored, and cut into thick slices

2 tablespoons olive oil

kosher salt to taste

6 cups chicken broth

1 russet potato, cut into 8 pieces

½ cup heavy whipping cream

1 pinch cayenne pepper

Instructions

Preheat the oven to 450 degrees F (230 degrees C). Line a baking sheet with aluminum foil.

Spread parsnips and apples out onto the prepared baking sheet. Drizzle olive oil over the top and sprinkle with kosher salt. Toss to coat.

Roast in the preheated oven until parsnips and apples are tender and caramelized around the edges, about 30 minutes.

Stir apple-parsnip mixture, chicken broth, and potato together in a large pot; bring to a boil, reduce heat to low, and simmer until potatoes are tender, about 30 minutes.

Purée apple mixture with an immersion blender until soup is smooth. Stir cream into soup and season with cayenne pepper and salt; cook until heated through, 2 to 5 minutes.

Stracciatella Soup

What You Need

6 cups chicken broth

salt and freshly ground black pepper to taste

3 large eggs

½ ounce grated Parmigiano-Reggiano cheese

½ ounce grated pecorino Romano cheese

2 tablespoons chopped fresh parsley

2 tablespoons semolina flour

1 pinch cayenne pepper

1 pinch freshly grated nutmeg

1 tablespoon olive oil

1 pinch red pepper flakes

Instructions

Bring broth to a simmer in a pot over high heat. Taste broth and adjust salt and pepper as needed.

Whisk eggs, grated Parmigiano Reggiano and Pecorino Romano cheeses, parsley, semolina flour, salt, pepper, cayenne, and nutmeg together in a bowl until well blended.

While stirring the simmering broth, slowly pour egg mixture into the broth. Bring mixture back up to a simmer. The liquid will be slightly cloudy initially and clear as broth heats.

Serve in bowls; garnish with a drizzle of olive oil and a pinch of red pepper flakes.

Feta Shrimp Soup

What You Need

1 tablespoon butter

2 tablespoons olive oil

1 medium onion, chopped

2 cloves garlic, minced

5 roma (plum) tomatoes, peeled and chopped

1 (8 ounce) bottle clam juice

1 cup dry white wine

¾ teaspoon dried oregano

1 pinch salt

½ teaspoon pepper

4 ounces crumbled feta cheese

1 pound medium shrimp - peeled and deveined

¼ cup chopped fresh parsley

Instructions

Melt the butter and heat the olive oil in a large pot over medium heat. Stir in the onion and garlic, and cook until tender. Mix in the tomatoes, clam juice, and wine. Season with oregano, salt, and pepper. Bring to a boil, reduce heat to low, and simmer 10 minutes.

Transfer soup in batches to a blender, and puree until smooth. Return to the pot, and stir in feta cheese. Continue cooking 10 minutes.

Stir the shrimp into the soup, and continue cooking 3 minutes, or until shrimp are opaque. Mix in parsley just before serving.

Zucchini Fenchel Suppe (Zucchini and Fennel Soup)

What You Need

2 tablespoons butter

1 onion, finely chopped

1 bulb fennel, diced, green tops reserved

1 zucchini, peeled and thinly sliced

2 cups chicken stock

1 teaspoon mild curry powder

salt and freshly ground black pepper to taste

1 teaspoon white wine vinegar, or to taste

Instructions

Melt butter in a large pot over medium heat. Add onion; cook and stir until softened, about 5 minutes. Add fennel bulb and zucchini; cook, stirring occasionally, for 3 minutes. Pour in chicken stock. Reduce heat to low and simmer soup, covered, until fennel is soft, 10 to 15 minutes.

Puree soup with an immersion blender until smooth. Season with curry powder, salt, and black pepper. Add white wine vinegar.

Chop reserved fennel tops finely and sprinkle over soup before serving.

Italian Sausage Soup

What You Need

1 pound Italian sausage

1 clove garlic, minced

2 (14 ounce) cans beef broth

1 (14.5 ounce) can Italian-style stewed tomatoes

1 cup sliced carrots

¼ teaspoon salt

¼ teaspoon ground black pepper

1 (14.5 ounce) can great Northern beans, undrained

2 small zucchini, cubed

2 cups spinach - packed, rinsed and torn

Instructions

Heat a stockpot or Dutch oven over medium-high heat. Add sausage and garlic; cook and stir until browned, 5 to 7 minutes. Stir in broth, tomatoes, and carrots; season with salt and pepper. Reduce heat to medium-low, cover, and simmer 15 minutes.

Stir in beans with liquid and zucchini; cover and simmer another 15 minutes, or until zucchini is tender.

Remove soup from heat and add spinach; replace the lid and allow spinach to wilt. Stir until warmed through.

Spanish Garlic Soup

What You Need

2 tablespoons olive oil

1 head garlic, peeled and lightly crushed

6 cups chicken stock

2 carrots, cut into matchsticks

1 red bell pepper, thinly sliced

salt and pepper to taste

Instructions

Heat oil in a large saucepan over medium heat. Stir in garlic and cook until lightly browned, about 5 minutes. Pour in 1 cup of chicken stock, cover, and allow to simmer until the garlic is soft, about 10 minutes.

Mash the garlic with a fork into a coarse paste. Pour in remaining chicken stock, increase heat to medium-high, and bring to a boil. Stir in carrots and cook for 1 minute, then add red pepper and continue cooking until vegetables are tender. Season to taste with salt and pepper before serving.

Asparagus, Lemon, and Mint Soup

What You Need

1 pound fresh asparagus, trimmed

1 tablespoon olive oil

1 shallot, chopped

1 tablespoon chopped fresh mint

sea salt and freshly ground black pepper to taste

2 cups chicken stock, or more if needed

1 teaspoon lemon zest

1 hard-boiled egg, chopped

Instructions

Cut tips from 6 asparagus spears, about 1 1/2 inches from the top; reserve for garnish later. Chop the remaining asparagus into chunks.

Heat olive oil in a soup pot over medium heat; cook and stir shallot in the hot oil until softened, about 3 minutes. Add chopped asparagus; season with mint, salt, and pepper. Cook until asparagus are slightly tender, about 3 minutes.

Pour chicken stock into asparagus mixture; bring to a boil. Reduce heat and simmer until asparagus are tender, 12 to 15 minutes. Stir in lemon zest.

Blend soup using a hand blender or a food processor until smooth.

Bring a small pot of lightly salted water to a boil; cook asparagus tips in the boiling water until just turning bright green, about 2 minutes. Strain asparagus tips and run under cold water to stop the cooking process. Garnish soup with asparagus tips and hard-boiled egg.

Fresh Asparagus Soup

What You Need

1 pound fresh asparagus

¾ cup chopped onion

½ cup vegetable broth

1 tablespoon butter

2 tablespoons all-purpose flour

1 teaspoon salt

1 pinch ground black pepper

1 ¼ cups vegetable broth

1 cup soy milk

½ cup yogurt

1 teaspoon lemon juice

¼ cup grated Parmesan cheese

Instructions

Place asparagus and onion in a saucepan with 1/2 cup vegetable broth. Bring the broth to a boil, reduce heat and let simmer until the vegetables are tender.

Reserve a few asparagus tips for garnish. Place remaining vegetable mixture in an electric blender and puree until smooth.

Melt butter in the pan that was used for simmering the asparagus and onions. Stir while sprinkling flour, salt, and pepper into the butter. Do not let the flour brown. Allow the mixture to cook only 2 minutes. Stir in remaining 1 1/4 cups vegetable broth and increase the heat. Continue stirring until the mixture comes to a boil.

Stir the vegetable puree and milk into the saucepan. Whisk yogurt into the mixture, followed by lemon juice. Stir until heated through, then ladle into bowls. Garnish with reserved asparagus tips. Sprinkle with Parmesan cheese if desired.

Southwestern Turkey Soup

What You Need

1 ½ cups shredded cooked turkey

4 cups vegetable broth

1 (28 ounce) can whole peeled tomatoes

1 (4 ounce) can chopped green chile peppers

2 roma (plum) tomatoes, chopped

1 onion, chopped

2 cloves garlic, crushed

1 tablespoon lime juice

½ teaspoon cayenne pepper

½ teaspoon ground cumin

salt and pepper to taste

1 avocado - peeled, pitted and diced

½ teaspoon dried cilantro

1 cup shredded Monterey Jack cheese

Instructions

In a large pot over medium heat, combine turkey, broth, canned tomatoes, green chiles, fresh tomatoes, onion, garlic, and lime juice. Season with cayenne, cumin, salt, and pepper. Bring to a boil, then reduce heat, and simmer 15 to 20 minutes.

Stir in avocado and cilantro, and simmer 15 to 20 minutes, until slightly thickened. Spoon into serving bowls, and top with shredded cheese.

Coconut Black Bean Soup

What You Need

2 (15 ounce) cans black beans, rinsed and drained

1 (14.5 ounce) can diced tomatoes

1 (14 ounce) can coconut milk

1 cup vegetable broth

2 green onions, chopped, or more to taste

1 tablespoon ground ginger

1 tablespoon ground cumin

1 tablespoon ground turmeric

2 cloves garlic, minced, or more to taste

salt to taste

Instructions

Combine black beans, tomatoes, coconut milk, broth, green onions, ginger, cumin, turmeric, and garlic in a large saucepan; bring to a boil. Reduce the heat and simmer until desired consistency is reached, 30 to 45 minutes. Season with salt.

Cheeseburger Soup

What You Need

4 tablespoons butter, divided

½ pound ground beef

¾ cup chopped onion

¾ cup shredded carrots

¾ cup chopped celery

1 teaspoon dried basil

1 teaspoon dried parsley

4 cups cubed potatoes

3 cups chicken broth

¼ cup all-purpose flour

1 ½ cups milk

2 cups cubed Cheddar cheese

¼ cup sour cream

Instructions

Melt 1 tablespoon butter in a large pot over medium heat; add ground beef, onion, carrots, and celery. Cook and stir until beef is browned and crumbly, 5 to 7 minutes.

Stir in basil and parsley. Add potatoes and broth and bring to a boil; reduce heat to low and simmer until potatoes are tender, 10 to12 minutes.

Melt remaining 3 tablespoons butter in a small saucepan over medium heat. Add flour and whisk until smooth, about 1 minute. Gradually whisk in milk; simmer and stir until sauce is thick and smooth.

Stir sauce into soup, stirring constantly. Bring to a boil; reduce heat to low and stir in cheese until melted. Add sour cream; stir until just heated through.

Serve hot and enjoy!

KIDNEY-SUPPORTIVE SWEET TREAT IDEAS

Lava Cake

What You Need

6 ½ (1 ounce) squares semisweet chocolate, finely chopped

½ cup butter, cut into 8 pieces

3 eggs, room temperature

⅓ cup white sugar

2 tablespoons all-purpose flour

4 teaspoons unsweetened cocoa powder

1 pinch salt

Instructions

Preheat the oven to 400 degrees F (200 degrees C). Grease and flour four 6-ounce ramekins.

Place chocolate and butter in the top of a double boiler over simmering water. Stir frequently, scraping down the sides with a rubber spatula to avoid scorching, until chocolate is melted, about 5 minutes.

Combine eggs and sugar in a large bowl; beat with an electric mixer until pale and thick, about 5 minutes. Mix in melted chocolate, flour, and cocoa powder until combined. Pour batter into the prepared ramekins and place on a baking tray.

Bake in the preheated oven until the sides are set but the middle is still jiggly, 10 to 13 minutes. Let cool for 5 minutes before serving.

Quiche Lorraine

What You Need

24 (3 inch) frozen tart shells, thawed

6 slices bacon, or more to taste

1 ¼ cups shredded Swiss cheese, divided (Optional)

2 green onions, diced

1 ¼ cups milk

4 large eggs

1 teaspoon Dijon mustard

¼ teaspoon salt

¼ teaspoon ground black pepper

Instructions

Preheat the oven to 375 degrees F (190 degrees C). Arrange tart shells in two 12-cup muffin tins; line each shell with a layer of pie weights or dried beans.

Bake in the preheated oven until crust edges are lightly browned and shells are about 3/4 fully cooked, 5 to 10 minutes. Remove from the oven and let sit until needed.

While the shells are baking, cook bacon in a large skillet over medium-high heat, turning occasionally, until browned and crispy, 7 to 10 minutes. Drain on paper towels and crumble when cooled.

Mix 1 cup Swiss, green onions, and crumbled bacon together in a bowl; divide mixture evenly among tart shells.

Whisk milk, eggs, mustard, salt, and pepper together in a bowl. Ladle egg mixture into each tart shell until about 2/3 full. Sprinkle remaining 1/4 cup Swiss over tarts.

Bake in the preheated oven until set in the middle and shells are golden brown, 25 to 30 minutes.

Mini Pecan Pies

What You Need

1 ½ cups pecan halves

1 cup white sugar

3 large eggs, beaten

½ cup light corn syrup

½ cup dark corn syrup

2 tablespoons butter, melted

1 teaspoon vanilla extract

¼ teaspoon salt

18 (3-inch) ready-to-bake pie shells

Instructions

Preheat the oven to 350 degrees F (175 degrees C).

Place pecans on a food processor and pulse until coarsely chopped.

Mix sugar, eggs, light corn syrup, dark corn syrup, butter, vanilla extract, and salt together in a bowl; fold in pecans. Spoon 1/4 cup pecan mixture into each mini pie shell. Transfer pies onto a baking sheet.

Bake in the preheated oven until mini pies are slightly browned, 25 to 30 minutes.

Meringues

What You Need

2 large egg whites

½ cup superfine sugar

1 teaspoon vanilla extract

Instructions

Preheat the oven to 300 degrees F (150 degrees C). Line a baking sheet with parchment paper.

Beat egg whites in a large bowl with an electric mixer until stiff, but not dry. Gradually beat in sugar until a little of the mixture between your thumb and forefinger feels smooth, not gritty. Stir in vanilla.

Pipe or spoon small portions onto the prepared baking sheet.

Bake in the preheated oven until dry but not brown, about 35 minutes. Turn the oven off and leave meringues inside to cool for at least 25 minutes.

Little Nut Cups

What You Need

1 cup butter, softened

2 (3 ounce) packages cream cheese

½ cup white sugar

2 cups all-purpose flour

2 teaspoons butter, melted

2 eggs

½ teaspoon vanilla extract

2 cups chopped pecans

1 ½ cups brown sugar

½ cup honey

Instructions

In a medium bowl, mix together the butter, cream cheese and sugar until smooth. Stir in the flour and mix thoroughly. The dough should be somewhat firm. Roll into 36 small balls, place them on a plate and refrigerate for one hour.

Make the filling in a medium bowl. Beat the eggs, melted butter, vanilla and brown sugar until smooth and well blended. Stir in the nuts. Preheat oven to 375 degrees F (190 degrees C). Press the chilled dough balls into the bottom and up the sides of tart pans or mini muffin cups. Fill each shell with filling almost to the top. Use a squeeze top honey container if you have one, to drip about 1/2 teaspoon of honey onto the top of each cup.

Bake for 15 to 20 minutes in the preheated oven, until crust is lightly browned. Allow to cool in the tins completely before removing.

Bologna Sliders with Fried Onions

What You Need

8 slider rolls

8 teaspoons yellow mustard

8 dill pickle slices, or more to taste

2 teaspoons olive oil

1 large onion, halved and thinly sliced

4 (1/4-inch-thick) slices deli bologna, quartered

Instructions

Slice slider rolls in half horizontally. Spread 1 teaspoon mustard on the bottom of each roll, top with a pickle slice, and set aside.

Heat 2 teaspoons olive oil in a large skillet over medium heat. Add sliced onions to skillet, cook for 1 minute and add the bologna wedges.

Cook until onions are tender and translucent, and the bologna is browned on each side, stirring and flipping occasionally, about 3 to 4 minutes.

Add 2 bologna wedges on top of each bottom bun and top with fried onions. Put tops of slider rolls back onto sliders; serve warm.

Baked Pumpkin Custard

What You Need

3 large eggs

1 cup 100% pure pumpkin

1 ½ teaspoons pumpkin pie spice

1 (14 ounce) can EAGLE BRAND® Sweetened Condensed Milk

1 ⅓ cups whole milk

1 teaspoon vanilla extract

¼ teaspoon salt

½ cup whipped cream, or to taste

1 pinch ground cinnamon, or to taste

Instructions

Preheat the oven to 350 degrees F (175 degrees C).

Whisk eggs together in a large bowl. Stir in pumpkin and pumpkin pie spice until blended. Whisk in condensed milk, milk, vanilla, and salt until blended. Pour into six 6-ounce custard cups.

Place custard cups in a 9x13-inch baking dish. Place the dish on the center rack in the middle of the preheated oven. Pour boiling water into the pan around custard cups to a depth of 1 1/4 inches.

Bake until the centers are almost set, about 35 minutes.

Remove custard cups from the baking dish and set on a wire rack to cool. Serve warm or cold. Top with whipped cream and sprinkle with cinnamon just before serving.

Cranberry Brie Bites

What You Need

1 (8 ounce) round Brie cheese

cooking spray

1 sheet frozen puff pastry, thawed

½ cup cranberry sauce

½ cup finely chopped walnuts

sea salt to taste

Instructions

Remove and discard rind from Brie cheese. Place cheese in the freezer for 20 minutes to make it easier to cut.

Meanwhile, oil a 24-cup mini muffin pan with cooking spray.

Roll puff pastry sheet out into a 10x14-inch rectangle. Cut sheet lengthwise into 4 even strips and then crosswise into 6 even strips, making 24 squares. Separate squares and gently press each one into a prepared muffin cup.

Remove chilled Brie from the freezer; cut into 24 pieces, approximately 3/4-inch in size.

Add 1 teaspoon cranberry sauce to each pastry-lined muffin cup, then press in a piece of Brie and top with 1 teaspoon chopped walnuts. Season each bite with a pinch of sea salt. Transfer muffin pan to the refrigerator and chill for at least 30 minutes, or cover and chill for up to 3 days.

When ready to bake, preheat the oven to 400 degrees F (200 degrees C).

Bake bites in the preheated oven until golden brown, 18 to 20 minutes.

Grilled Hot Dog Sliders

What You Need

8 bun-length long hot dogs (such as Sabrett Skinless Frankfurters) or 12 regular hot dogs

2 (12-pack packages) King's Hawaiian Rolls

assorted toppings (such as ketchup, mustard, relish, kraut, chili, cheese, and onions)

Instructions

Use a large serrated knife to slice the tops of each roll horizontally, taking care not to cut all the way through.

Preheat an outdoor grill for medium heat and lightly oil the grate.

Cook hot dogs to desired degree of doneness, 5 to 7 minutes. Remove from heat and cut hot dogs in thirds (if using the bun length hot dogs) or in half (if using regular size hot dogs). Place each hot dog in the cut centers of each roll and pull each roll apart to separate each hot dog. Serve with desired toppings.

Butter Tarts

What You Need

30 (2 inch) unbaked tart shells

1 ½ cups packed brown sugar

½ cup butter

2 eggs

2 cups raisins

1 cup chopped walnuts

2 tablespoons heavy cream

Instructions

Preheat the oven to 325 degrees F (170 degrees C). Arrange tart shells on a baking sheet.

Beat sugar, butter, and eggs together in a large bowl with an electric mixer until creamy.

Stir in raisins, walnuts, and cream until thoroughly combined. Spoon batter into tart shells, no more than half full.

Bake tarts in the preheated oven until pastry is golden and filling is set, 20 to 25 minutes. Allow tarts to cool on a wire rack.

Pepperoni Pizza Muffins

What You Need

cooking spray

1 (10 ounce) can refrigerated buttermilk biscuit dough

10 tablespoons pizza sauce (such as Ragu® Homestyle)

10 slices pepperoni

10 tablespoons shredded mozzarella cheese, or as needed

Instructions

Preheat the oven to 425 degrees F (220 degrees C). Spray 10 muffin cups with cooking spray. Press biscuits, one at a time, between hands to flatten. Place each flattened biscuit in a muffin cup; press into bottom and up sides of cup. Set aside for dough to settle and slightly rise, about

5 minutes; lightly press dough into cups if needed.

Spoon 1 tablespoon pizza sauce into each dough cup; top each with 1 slice pepperoni and 1 tablespoon mozzarella cheese.

Bake in the preheated oven until pizza muffins are lightly browned and cheese is melted, about 10 minutes. Remove from tin and place on a cooling rack to cool slightly, about 5 minutes.

Red Lobster Cheddar Biscuits

What You Need

2 cups all-purpose flour

1 cup shredded Cheddar cheese

1 tablespoon baking powder

1 teaspoon salt

½ teaspoon garlic powder

⅔ cup milk

⅓ cup butter, softened and cut into pieces

1 large egg

2 tablespoons butter, melted

2 teaspoons dried parsley (Optional)

1 teaspoon garlic powder (Optional)

Instructions

Preheat the oven to 400 degrees F (200 degrees C). Grease or line a baking sheet with parchment paper.

Stir flour, Cheddar cheese, baking powder, salt, and garlic powder together in a bowl.

Stir milk, softened butter pieces, and egg together in a separate bowl. Add to the flour mixture and stir until just combined and chunky, being very careful not to overmix.

Drop batter by tablespoonfuls onto the prepared baking sheet.

Bake in the preheated oven for 10 minutes.

Meanwhile, stir melted butter, parsley, and garlic powder together in a small bowl. Remove biscuits from the oven and brush melted butter mixture over top.

Return to the oven and bake until golden brown, about 5 more minutes. Serve warm.

Cake Pops

What You Need

1 (15.25 ounce) package yellow cake mix (such as Betty Crocker®)

1 cup water

3 large eggs

½ cup vegetable oil

1 (16 ounce) container prepared chocolate frosting

18 lollipop sticks

1 (14 ounce) bag chocolate candy melts

1 (.75 ounce) tube decorating icing

1 tablespoon multicolored candy sprinkles, or as needed (Optional)

Instructions

Preheat the oven to 350 degrees F (175 degrees C). Grease a 9x13-inch baking dish.

Beat cake mix, water, oil, and eggs in a bowl using an electric mixer on low speed for 30 seconds. Increase speed to medium and beat for 2 minutes more.

Pour batter into the prepared baking dish.

Bake in the preheated oven until a toothpick inserted in the center comes out clean, 28 to 33 minutes. Remove from the oven and cool completely, at least 1 hour.

Crumble cooled cake into a large bowl.

Stir frosting into the crumbled cake until mixture is sticky and starts to come together but is not too smooth. Refrigerate until chilled, for at least 30 minutes.

Roll cake mixture into eighteen 1 1/2-inch balls and place on a baking sheet.

Place about 1/4 cup candy melts in a microwave-safe bowl. Microwave on high until melted, about 20 seconds.

Push a lollipop stick halfway into each ball of cake mixture.

Gently dip balls into the melted chocolate to coat, then place upright in a block of styrofoam.

Decorate with candy sprinkles while chocolate coating is wet. Repeat to make remaining cake pops, melting more candy melts as needed.

Enjoy!

Red, White, and Blue Cheesecake Bites

What You Need

Crumb Crust:

1/2 cup finely crushed graham cracker crumbs

1 tablespoon white sugar

2 tablespoons melted butter

1/8 teaspoon vanilla extract

Cheesecake:

1 pound cream cheese, at room temperature

1 lime, zested

1/2 cup white sugar

1/2 teaspoon vanilla extract

1 tablespoon all-purpose flour

2 large eggs

Whipped Topping and Fruit:

1/2 cup cold heavy cream

1 tablespoon sour cream

24 slices fresh strawberry

72 fresh blueberries

Instructions

Preheat the oven to 325 degrees F (165 degrees C). Spray 2 12-cup mini muffin tins with nonstick cooking spray, and use your finger to make sure the inside of each cup is well greased. Place muffin tins on a sheet pan.

Stir together graham cracker crumbs, 1 tablespoon sugar, butter, and 1/8 teaspoon vanilla extract in a bowl until crumb mixture resembles wet sand. Spoon a slightly rounded teaspoon of crumb mixture into the bottom of each cup. Use a spoon to spread crumbs into a relatively even layer.

Set one muffin pan on top of the other and press lightly to compact the crumbs. Repeat with the other pan.

Combine softened cream cheese, lime zest, and 1/2 cup sugar in a bowl, and beat until light and fluffy with an electric mixer or whisk. Add 1/2 teaspoon vanilla, flour, and 1 egg; beat until egg is incorporated and mixture is smooth. Add remaining egg; whisk until smooth.

Transfer batter into a piping bag, and pipe into the muffin tins, filling them all the way to the top. You can use a spoon; but a piping bag is neater and takes much less time. Use a skewer to stir each cup to remove any air bubbles. Tap pan on the counter to settle batter down.

Bake in the preheated oven until batter rises slightly and very small cracks appear on the surface, 20 to 25 minutes. The cheesecakes on the inside may cook more slowly than the ones on the outside, and may not rise as high or crack.

Let cool to room temperature, about 20 minutes. Remove from the tins. Wrap and refrigerate cheesecakes until fully chilled, at least 30 minutes.

To make whipped cream topping, whisk cold cream in a bowl until soft peaks start to form. Add sour cream, and continue whisking until medium-stiff peaks form. Top each cold cheesecake with whipped cream, 3 blueberries, and 1 strawberry slice.

Baked Ham and Cheese Sliders

What You Need

¾ cup melted butter

1 ½ tablespoons Dijon mustard

1 ½ teaspoons Worcestershire sauce

1 ½ tablespoons poppy seeds

1 tablespoon dried minced onion

24 mini sandwich rolls

1 pound thinly sliced cooked deli ham

1 pound thinly sliced Swiss cheese

Instructions

Gather all What You Need.

Preheat the oven to 350 degrees F (175 degrees C). Grease a 9x13-inch baking dish.

Mix butter, Dijon mustard, Worcestershire sauce, poppy seeds, and dried onion in a bowl.

Separate the tops from the bottoms of the rolls; arrange the bottom pieces in a layer in the prepared baking dish. Layer about 1/2 of the ham onto the rolls; add a layer of Swiss cheese and top with remaining ham slices.

Place the tops of the rolls onto the sandwiches. Pour mustard mixture evenly over the rolls Bake in the preheated oven until the rolls are lightly browned and the cheese has melted, about 20 minutes. Slice into individual rolls through the ham and cheese layers to serve.

CHAPTER V: FINAL NOTES

Individuals diagnosed with chronic kidney disease (CKD) often discover that adopting dietary modifications can significantly enhance their overall well-being. Collaborating with a certified dietitian is paramount in crafting a personalized diet regimen that not only promotes optimal kidney health but also ensures a satisfying culinary experience.

One pivotal aspect of managing CKD entails prioritizing meals with reduced salt and sodium content to effectively regulate blood pressure. It's advisable to adhere to a daily salt intake of no more than 2,300 mg, a measure that can be facilitated by embracing fresh, home-cooked meals. Unlike their processed and restaurant counterparts, which often harbor elevated sodium levels, homemade dishes offer greater control over ingredient composition.

In navigating the culinary landscape, it's crucial to discern between foods that naturally contain minimal salt and those that are laden with it. Packaged goods typically bear Nutrition Facts labels, serving as invaluable tools in assessing sodium concentrations. Aim for products boasting designations such as "sodium-free," "salt-free," "low-sodium," "reduced-sodium," "no salt," or "lightly salted" to guide your selections. Additionally, scrutinizing the Daily Value percentage can help identify high-sodium items, with figures exceeding 20% signaling a need for caution.

Exploring alternative flavoring agents, such as herbs, spices, and seasonings, can enrich the taste profile of dishes sans excessive sodium. Furthermore, when resorting to convenience items like frozen meals or canned goods, opt for those with lower salt content. Prior to consumption, rinsing canned vegetables, beans, meats, and fish under water can mitigate their sodium levels, contributing to a healthier dietary regimen.

Maintaining an appropriate balance of protein is imperative, as excessive protein consumption can potentially strain the kidneys due to the metabolic byproducts generated. Consulting with a dietitian to ascertain the optimal quantity and quality of protein intake is advisable, ensuring that dietary choices align with both kidney health requirements and personal preferences.

By conscientiously navigating food choices and embracing a culinary approach that prioritizes kidney health without compromising on enjoyment, individuals with CKD can embark on a journey toward enhanced well-being and vitality.

www.ingramcontent.com/pod-product-compliance
Lightning Source LLC
Chambersburg PA
CBHW052248220526
45471CB00001B/244